The Asthma Sourcebook

Francis V. Adams, M.D.

McGraw Hill

New York Chicago San Francisco Lisbon London Madrid Mexico City
Milan New Delhi San Juan Seoul Singapore Sydney Toronto

The McGraw·Hill Companies

Library of Congress Cataloging-in-Publication Data

Adams, Francis V.
    The asthma sourcebook / Francis V. Adams. — 3rd ed.
        p.   cm.
    Includes bibliographical references and index.
    ISBN 0-07-147652-0 (alk. paper)
    1. Asthma—Popular works.   I. Title.

    RC591.A325   2007
    616.2'38—dc22   2006022980

1 2 3 4 5 6 7 8 9 10 11 12 13 14 15   DOC/DOC   0 9 8 7 6

ISBN-13: 978-0-07-147652-2
ISBN-10:   0-07-147652-0

McGraw-Hill books are available at special quantity discounts to use as premiums and sales
promotions, or for use in corporate training programs. For more information, please write to
the Director of Special Sales, Professional Publishing, McGraw-Hill, Two Penn Plaza, New York,
NY 10121-2298. Or contact your local bookstore.

Also by Francis V. Adams, M.D.
The Breathing Disorders Sourcebook
Healing Through Empathy

This book is printed on acid-free paper.

In memory of Dr. Loren Tierney, who gave light from her eyes, empathy through her voice, and healing with her touch

For MEK

Contents

Preface

IN THE PAST two decades, our understanding of the genetic and chemical nature of asthma has increased tremendously. Based on this emerging information, scientists are now poised to produce targeted treatments for individuals who are susceptible to asthma. In the next century asthma treatments are likely to alter the course of the disease and possibly prevent its occurrence.

Despite many exciting advances, the number of asthma cases has again increased after a brief decline. Asthma is still "the silent epidemic" of the inner city. The prevalence of childhood asthma in North America remains among the world's highest. The effects of this health care crisis are felt throughout our society through sudden deaths, disability, increased expenditures, and lost productivity.

Why is asthma again on the rise? One of the most alarming aspects of the explosion in asthma cases in the last two decades is that there is no certain answer. It is likely that a combination of factors may explain this dramatic increase. Children are spending more time indoors, breathing in allergens that sensitize them to asthma. Although air pollution levels in the United States are lower, there are greater numbers of vehicles on the roads producing exhaust fumes, which, combined with pollution from other countries, have increased asthmatic reactions. Thirty percent of this nation's ozone, an important component of smog, and 40 percent of the air's mercury come from other nations.

Asthma is now regarded as a complex condition that occurs when a susceptible individual is exposed to environmental irritants. Ongoing research continues to produce large amounts of new information for physicians and patients. Paralleling this increase in information has been the expanded use of the Internet as a health information resource.

The Asthma Sourcebook was originally written to increase understanding of asthma and to encourage asthmatics to be active participants in their care. This third edition continues to achieve these goals by incorporating the most current information. Since the publication of the second edition of *The Asthma Sourcebook* in 1998, researchers have discovered several asthma genes and described their action, opening a new avenue of future treatments. A new test for the diagnosis and management of asthma, the NIOX Nitric Oxide Test System, was recently approved by the Food and Drug Administration (FDA). An entirely new asthma medication, omalizumab (Xolair), which blocks Immunoglobulin E (IgE), has been introduced. A second long-acting bronchodilator, formoterol (Foradil), as well as a new short-acting agent, levalbuterol (Xopenex), also have been added. A new inhaled corticosteroid, mometasone (Asmanex), is also available. The delivery system for many asthma medications has also changed with the use of a non-chlorofluorocarbon aerosol and single or multidose dry powder inhalers. At the same time that we have seen exciting advances in treatment, controversy regarding possible adverse effects of long-acting bronchodilators has increased.

In this edition of *The Asthma Sourcebook*, I have updated each chapter with the latest information available. In view of increasing interest in unorthodox therapies, Chapter 12 on alternative forms of treatment for asthma has been expanded. Chapter 13 (Future Considerations) has been revised to reflect the many exciting developments that we may expect in the coming years. The Appendix has been completely revised and updated with extensive Internet resources. This book is intended to provide important information for patients and their families as a supplement to their medical care. It is my hope that this updated edition will continue to be a valuable source of helpful information.

Introduction

ASTHMA IS A common disease that affects nearly 15 percent of the population in the United States, as many as twenty-one million Americans, and more than three hundred million people worldwide. Since asthma is often a mild illness, these numbers probably underestimate the true number of cases. A recent survey estimated that thirty-one million Americans had been diagnosed with asthma by a health professional within their lifetime. After a long period of steady increase, asthma rates declined from 1997 to 1999, but rates in 2000 and 2001 indicate a rising trend. In 2001, the cost of illness related to asthma was estimated at $14 billion. The source of the marked increase in asthma rates in the last two decades is not entirely clear. Air pollution has been implicated since the majority of asthmatics live in areas where pollution levels are high. Indoor pollution may also be a factor because windowless offices and airtight homes reduce air circulation, thus exposing asthmatics to higher levels of irritating substances.

The increase in asthma has been particularly striking in children, African Americans, Hispanics, and women. The greatest increase in asthma between 1997 and 2001 has been in children five to seventeen years of age. One out of three asthmatics in the United States is under eighteen years of age. In 2001, four million children had an asthma attack. Asthma appears to be most severe among black children, and blacks are three times as likely as whites to be hospitalized for treatment of asthma. In 2002, more than 1.7 million Hispanic Americans reported that they currently have asthma. Puerto Ricans have higher rates of asthma than other Hispanic subgroups and non-Hispanic whites. Women tend to have a consistently higher risk of having an asthmatic attack than men. In contrast to the increasing rates of asthma in the United States, hospitalizations and deaths due to asthma have declined, suggesting a better level of disease management. In 2000, 4,487 people died of asthma. Approximately 65 percent of these deaths occurred in women.

Several factors may explain these changes. In the last decade significant advances have improved our understanding of asthma. Even the definition of *asthma* has changed during this period. Asthma is now reclassified as an inflammatory process that occurs when a susceptible individual is exposed to a "pro-asthma environment." Besides greater understanding of the disease, physicians are now armed with a number of new medications that have improved the treatment and management of asthma. In this period two new classes of medication, the anti-leukotrienes and anti-IgE monoclonal antibody, have become available to patients in the United States. Genetic research has also determined that certain individuals may benefit more than others from asthma medications. Future asthma treatments will likely be "targeted" to provide the best possible results.

This book's goal is to educate asthmatics in order to improve their quality of life. Knowledge is essential to the beneficial management of asthma, and education continues to be sorely needed. For example, studies have shown that flu vaccine is safe to administer to adults and children with asthma, including those with severe asthma. Yet, fewer than 10 percent of patients with asthma currently receive the flu vaccine. If the percentage increased to only 50 percent, then close to 95,000 hospitalizations would be prevented and 530 million dollars saved per year.

A patient must first accept the presence of the disease, and then take an active role in its treatment. Too often patients' denial of their illnesses leads to more frequent and more severe asthmatic attacks. Asthma symptoms may be monitored at home with a peak flow meter, which encourages patients to participate in their own treatment. A well-informed patient is more likely to seek medical advice before an attack becomes severe. Improved communication between patients and physicians usually leads to formation of a "partnership" that helps to achieve better asthma management.

This book also should be helpful for friends and families of asthma patients. If others gain greater knowledge of the disease, they may be encouraged to provide vital support and better understanding. The value of support groups, including asthma camps, has been well documented.

Fatal asthma continues to occur when patients are either mistakenly diagnosed, are diagnosed too late, or do not seek medical attention. These deaths are especially tragic, since treatment can be lifesaving if given early and correctly. I hope this book will allow some patients to recognize they may have asthma and direct them to an appropriate caregiver. Those who have been diagnosed may learn how to better assess the severity of their illness and to plan how they will respond to an attack. In this way a greater number of asthmatic attacks may be recognized and treated before they become severe or prove fatal.

All patients should seek information from their physicians. This book is meant to be used as a supplement that hopefully will add useful information. Patients should know their disease and feel free to ask questions to increase their understanding. The Appendix contains additional suggestions for obtaining more information.

In my experience some of the most useful information comes from patient-initiated discussion, and much of the information in this book comes from listening to patients with asthma. I also have been privileged to study with a number of chest specialists who taught and encouraged me to pursue my practice of chest medicine. As a teenager I followed my father, Dr. Vincent J. Adams, on house calls and hospital rounds and saw firsthand what being a physician meant. When I was sixteen, my father taught me to do pulmonary function tests as well as the basics of their interpretation, which I continue to use in my own practice. At a young age I learned from him that you had to know and treat patients as individuals, not just as diseases.

When I was a medical student at Cornell, Drs. James Smith and Elliot Hochstein encouraged my interest in chest disease. At Georgetown University Hospital, Dr. Sol Katz embodied what a diagnostician of chest diseases should be. Finally, on the Bellevue

Chest Service three of the "giants" of chest medicine, Drs. John McClement, H. William Harris, and Lynn Christianson completed my formal chest education. The knowledge I gained from these gifted physicians and from thirty years of "hands-on" experience treating chest diseases provided the foundation for this book.

My opinions and recommendations represent my own approach to the treatment of bronchial asthma and should be so regarded. Controversies and differences of opinion permeate every aspect of medicine and asthma is no exception.

I am indebted to many for their assistance in preparing this text but can only mention a few. The medical illustrations were done by Laurel H. Adams. The photographs for Figures 2.1, 2.2, 3.3, 4.4, and 4.5 were done by Linda Covello. Mary Kane has worked tirelessly on all three editions of this book and has provided many helpful suggestions as well as extensive research and material for publication. My wife, Laura Anne, encouraged me to update this book even though she knew it would take many hours away from our precious time together. Bud Sperry of Lowell House first brought this project to my attention and enlisted my participation. Michele Matrisciani, Sarah Pelz, and Deborah Brody of McGraw-Hill made this third edition possible and worked to bring it to completion. I am grateful for this opportunity and hope this book will continue to prove useful to many.

Until I feared I would lose it, I never loved to read. One does not love breathing.

HARPER LEE, *TO KILL A MOCKINGBIRD*

1

What Is Asthma?

To UNDERSTAND ASTHMA you must first consider the normal structure of the lung. We will define *asthma* and discuss its causes as well as describe how a physician begins to make a diagnosis.

The Normal Lung

In a normal lung, two systems coexist to permit its function of enriching the blood with oxygen and excreting carbon dioxide. Oxygen is the fuel for metabolism while carbon dioxide represents the waste product.

The Bronchial Tubes

The first system is a series of hollow connecting airways that form the bronchial tubes. Imagine that this system resembles a large branching tree with the trunk being the windpipe (trachea) that begins below the voice box (larynx). Figure 1.1 shows the windpipe branching into two major bronchial divisions. Branching of this bronchial "tree" occurs frequently to the smallest imaginable airway, a bronchiole. The inner lining of the bronchial tubes is a delicate membrane called the bronchial mucosa. Although normally pale and innocent in appearance, this membrane is capable

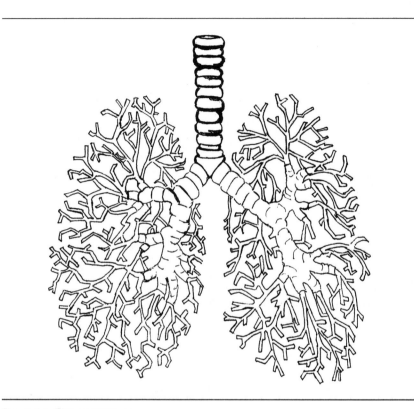

Figure 1.1 The normal lung

of becoming inflamed and swollen in an asthmatic attack. Mucous glands within the layers of the bronchial lining can produce large quantities of extremely thick secretion when stimulated by infection or asthma triggers. In the wall of the bronchial tubes is a smooth muscle layer capable of contracting, producing narrowing (bronchoconstriction), and capable of relaxing, producing widening (bronchodilatation).

The Alveoli

The second system within the lung consists of millions of tiny air sacs, or alveoli. Think of these sacs surrounding the small bronchial tubes like grapes surrounding a stem. In Figure 1.2 a bronchiole is surrounded by alveoli. Each of the smallest bronchioles allows air to enter and leave multiple alveoli. Within these small air sacs, the vital gas exchange takes place. Within the wall of these sacs, blood courses within small vessels called capillaries. This blood has been returned from all parts of the body where it has been used for metabolism. As it enters the capillaries, it is low in oxygen and high in carbon dioxide. The extremely thin walls of these blood vessels allow the exchange of oxygen and carbon dioxide. The blood leaves the alveoli rich in oxygen and lower in carbon dioxide.

The Nervous System and the Lung

Besides reviewing the normal structure of the lung, it is important to understand the role of the nervous system and how it relates to

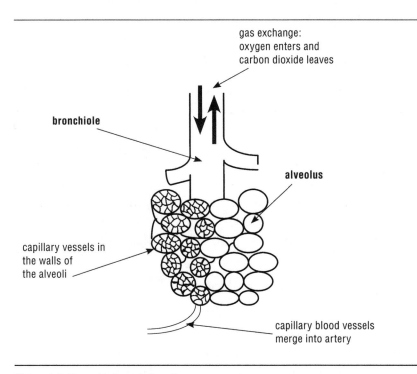

Figure 1.2 Bronchiole and alveoli

bronchial asthma. The nervous system is generally divided into the central structures of the brain and spinal cord and peripheral nerve structures distributed throughout the body.

The Autonomic Nervous System

One major subdivision of the nervous system is called the autonomic nervous system, which is responsible for the unconscious control of major body functions and is divided into a parasympathetic and a sympathetic branch. These systems extend throughout the body but are extremely important in lung function. Just think of these two systems as balancing each other. For example, stimulating the parasympathetic system causes the bronchial tubes to constrict while stimulating the sympathetic nervous system produces the opposite reaction (dilatation). In a normal lung a balance of these two systems maintains open airways. In an asthmatic lung, an imbalance occurs, favoring the parasympathetic system that produces narrowing, or constriction, of the air tubes.

Adrenergic Versus Cholinergic Effects

The effects produced through the nerve pathways are mediated by chemicals called neurotransmitters. These chemicals act at nerve endings or receptor sites throughout the body. In the parasympathetic nervous system, the neurotransmitter is a chemical substance known as acetylcholine. Agents or medications that mimic the effects of this substance are called cholinergic agents. In the sympathetic nervous system, the neurotransmitter is a substance known as epinephrine, or adrenaline. Agents or medications that mimic the effects of adrenaline are called adrenergic agents.

Receptors: Alpha and Beta

It is important to familiarize yourself with the different types of receptors that exist in the nerve endings. These receptors are divided into alphas and betas based on how they respond to medication. In general, alpha receptors excite and beta receptors usually inhibit or relax. Alpha receptors seem to be less important in regulating bronchial tubes than beta receptors. Beta receptors are classified as β_1, found in the heart muscle, and β_2, found in the bronchial tubes and other parts of the body. The effect of asthma medications on these receptors is discussed in Chapter 4.

Definition of *Asthma*

That asthma has been defined in so many ways reflects the complexity of this illness. As shown in Figure 1.3, several features of asthma, including reversible airway obstruction, inflammation, and hyperirritability, are covered by the currently accepted definition.

Airway Obstruction: Reversible

First, the airways of the lung or bronchial tubes are narrowed. This is called "airway obstruction" since air can no longer flow smoothly through this elaborate system of branching tubes. Since these tubes can dilate, or open, in asthma this obstruction is called reversible, an important aspect of the definition since it may distinguish asthma from other bronchial illnesses with fixed or irreversible obstruction such as bronchitis and emphysema.

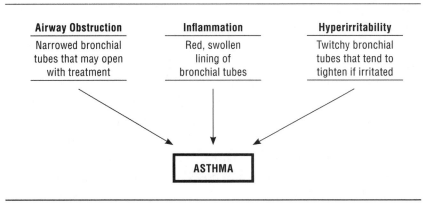

Figure 1.3 Definition of asthma

This narrowing within the bronchial tubes has occurred due to a tightening or constriction of the muscle that exists in the bronchial wall. This reaction may be thought of as a muscle "spasm" that results in narrowing of the bronchial tubes, similar to any muscle cramp. It is these narrowed or "obstructed" airways that produce one of the common features of asthma, the wheeze. As air is exhaled through these tubes, its movement is turbulent and produces this sound.

Inflammation

The second element included in defining *asthma* is the presence of inflammation, the red, swollen appearance of the inside of the bronchial tubes. This characteristic of asthma has received a great deal of attention and has become the focus of much of asthma research and therapy. The inflammation is present in the lining (the mucosa) of the bronchial tubes, which can be examined by inserting into them a lighted scope called a bronchoscope. With this instrument a physician can also obtain samples of the bronchial lining and its secretions. Under a microscope these samples may show large numbers of cells that carry substances called mediators capable of causing inflammation. Using these techniques, the asthma mediators released by inflammatory cells when an attack occurs can be measured and identified. Microscopic samples of the bronchial lining in asthma patients also show swelling and thickening of this tissue, often referred to as "remodeling" of the bronchial mucosa.

Hyperirritability

The third defining feature is increased responsiveness, or hyperirritability, of the bronchial tubes and their tendency to "overreact" and narrow. The term "twitchy" has also been used in this regard. This irritability is often demonstrated by the sudden, severe attacks patients can experience when exposed to substances such as pollen, animal dander, dust, and fumes. This hyperreactivity forms the basis for bronchial provocation or challenge testing that is used by physicians to diagnose asthma in patients whose illnesses do not fit easily into the other defining features.

What Causes Asthma?

The development of asthma is now believed to result from an interaction between a susceptible individual and the environment. Something in the environment "presses" on specific genes to cause asthma to appear. Several factors are involved in this complex process. (See Figure 1.4.)

Heredity

Heredity plays a major role in the development of asthma, as asthma and allergy often occur in families. Asthma is more common in certain regions and populations around the world. Individuals who are susceptible to asthma appear to have inherited specific genes for allergy, asthma, and bronchial hyperresponsiveness.

Geneticists have estimated that there are as many as ten genes that have a significant effect on a person's susceptibility to asthma. About half of these genes have already been identified. A gene called ADAM33 located on chromosome 20 appears to play a crucial role in making the bronchial tubes oversensitive or hyperresponsive, increasing the risk of asthma. A recently discovered asthma gene, called PHF11, is located on chromosome 13, which for many years has been known to contain an asthma gene, until now unspecified. This gene appears to regulate blood cells that produce Immuno-globulin E (IgE), an allergic protein that has the ability to "lock on" the surface of allergy cells called mast cells. When IgE reacts with allergy substances known as allergens, the mast cell disin-tegrates, releasing irritating chemicals that cause inflammation. These chemicals are the asthma mediators. By identifying PHF11, scientists may now target this gene with drugs that could turn off IgE production and prevent allergic disease. In the next few years it is likely that all of the remaining genes involved in asthma will be identified, presenting scientists with information from which new treatments will be developed.

The Immune System

The immune system also plays a major role in the development of asthma. The immune system has two basic branches: cellular and humoral. Cellular immunity involves white blood cells called lymphocytes that can be provoked, or "sensitized." An example of this would be the body's rejection process against a transplanted organ. Humoral immunity involves the production of substances called antibodies and immunoglobulin that circulate in the blood. An example would be how the body reacts to a vaccination by producing antibodies. An antigen (may also be called an allergen) is a substance capable of provoking the immune response. When allergens enter the body, they are engulfed by scavenger cells called macrophages. These activated cells stimulate both cellular and humoral responses that ultimately produce an allergic and/or asthmatic reaction.

Lymphocytes, Mast Cells, and Eosinophils. In asthma, the immune system is provoked in two ways. First, the cellular elements are mobilized and activated. Microscopic studies of the lining of the bronchial tubes in asthma have revealed increased numbers of lymphocytes. These cells produce substances that result in an increase in the number of mast cells that are known to store and release many irritating chemicals involved in production of the asthmatic reaction. These chemical substances, or mediators of asthma, produce inflammation. Another active cell that is "recruited" by lymphocytes found in the inflamed bronchial lining is the eosinophil. Large numbers of these cells may also be found in the blood of allergic and asthmatic individuals.

Immunoglobulin E. The second major immune response in allergy and asthma is the production of antibodies known as

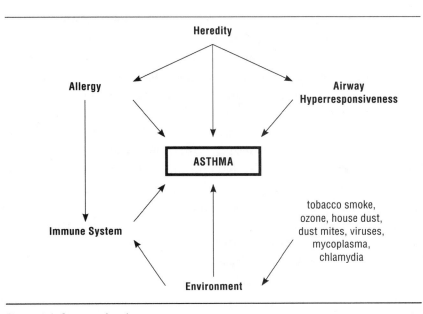

Figure 1.4 Causes of asthma

immunoglobulins, which is stimulated by substances released by the activated lymphocytes. In an allergic person, one type, Immunoglobulin E (IgE), may be produced by inhaling a specific allergen such as ragweed. When the ragweed-activated IgE attaches to the surface of the mast cell and combines with ragweed particles, the cell is punctured, releasing "asthma chemicals" that produce an asthmatic reaction.

Allergy

Allergy, an abnormal reaction or increased sensitivity to certain substances, is the leading cause of asthma. In allergic patients allergens, activated lymphocytes, mast cells, eosinophils, and IgE all play major roles in the immune response that produces the asthmatic reaction. However, asthma also may occur without allergy. In nonallergic patients doctors believe the immune response that leads to asthma may be triggered by infection.

The most common allergens are animal danders, pollens, house dust, dust mites, molds, foods (shellfish, nuts, and dairy products), medications, and insect bites. Allergic reactions may take many forms but most commonly involve the nose (hay fever) and bronchial tubes (asthma). In children, the constant upward wiping of the dripping allergic nose has been called the "allergy salute."

Other parts of the body may also have allergic reactions. In the eye, allergy commonly causes inflammation of the lining of the eyelid known as conjunctivitis. This produces itching, which leads to frequent rubbing. Allergy may affect the skin in several forms. In eczema, rashes develop, accompanied by severe itching. This may occur in infants, commonly on the face and later inside the elbows and backs of the knees or on the ankles, wrists, or hands. Another common allergic skin condition is hives (urticaria) in which red, itchy, raised blotches appear.

Who May Become Allergic? The greatest risk of developing allergy comes from having an allergic parent. Children of allergic parents, however, may never develop allergies, and allergic children may be born to nonallergic parents. It is clear from this information that other factors, such as the environment, infections, and repeated exposure to allergens, play a strong role in the development of allergy.

Viruses, Chlamydia, and Mycoplasma

Viral infections in susceptible individuals have been thought to be potent triggers for the development of asthma. Researchers have demonstrated that viruses may cause human immune system cells to produce IgE. Animal research has shown that viruses are capable of altering the nervous impulses that stimulate the bronchial tubes. The altered nerve impulses may then produce constriction in the bronchial tubes. Susceptible patients with viral bronchial infections may become "sensitized" and display all the features noted in the defining features of asthma.

Two additional infectious agents, chlamydia and mycoplasma, have been found in large numbers of asthmatics and are strongly implicated in the development of both sudden as well as chronic asthma. In many of these patients, the treatment of these infections with antibiotics may have a favorable effect on controlling the asthma.

The Environment

The development of asthma may be determined by the interaction between a susceptible individual and the environment. Exposure early in life to allergens, cigarette smoke, infections, pollutants (ozone or particulates), dust, chemicals, and proteins may set the stage for the development of chronic asthma. Environmental irritants also account for large numbers of asthmatic attacks each year and may explain an increase in the number of asthma cases, especially in large cities.

The Future

In the last two decades promising research has shown that asthma is an inflammatory disease. A large number of specific chemical substances or mediators involved in the asthmatic reaction have been identified, leading to the development of medications that inhibit or block the action of these chemicals. During this same time period, the "genetic code" for asthma has been broken. Future treatments of asthma are likely to result from these two avenues of research.

Extrinsic Versus Intrinsic Asthma

Asthma is often divided into either an allergic, or "extrinsic," type that commonly has its onset in childhood and an adult-onset, or "intrinsic," type. Although there is considerable overlap between these groups, it is helpful to classify patients according to several features that distinguish them.

Extrinsic Asthma

Extrinsic patients are younger and have attacks clearly triggered by exposure to allergens such as pollens, dust, animal dander, foods, and molds. These patients often have strong family histories of relatives with allergies or asthma. Allergy treatment known as desensitization has often been helpful in these patients. For many years it has been thought that the majority of these patients "outgrew" their asthma by age thirty, but recent evidence suggests that 75 percent remain asthmatic for life. These patients may have long symptom-free periods.

Intrinsic Asthma

Intrinsic patients often develop asthma as adults, and at any age. Often the trigger for these attacks is infection with involvement of the lower respiratory tract as in bronchitis or pneumonia. Some of the most severe infections of this type are viral, but they also may be due to bacteria or other agents such as chlamydia or mycoplasma. Patients in the intrinsic group usually do not have histories of allergies and produce negative allergy tests. Once the diagnosis is evident, further attacks are often triggered by less severe infections. There are fewer symptom-free periods in this group, and these patients usually require medication for life.

Should This Classification Be Used?

Many practitioners no longer use this older classification of the types of bronchial asthma. When discussing the future outlook of the disease as well as treatment options, I find it helpful to use these two general classes of asthma to provide simple guidelines that can be followed. In the younger, highly allergic, or extrinsic asthmatic, for example, emphasis on avoidance of allergens will be extremely important. Less time would be spent discussing this topic for patients with intrinsic asthma with greater emphasis on the prevention and treatment of respiratory infections.

How Is the Diagnosis of Asthma Made?
The Medical History

All diagnoses begin with a thorough medical history. The physician looks for the age at onset of symptoms and associated allergies. Evidence of airway obstruction may be suggested by a report of wheezing and shortness of breath. Coughing may be a prominent symptom and the physician will inquire as to the character of phlegm produced. The physician will also ask about the presence of nasal symptoms, sinus pain, or infection as well as the presence of allergic skin problems such as rash (eczema) or hives (urticaria). A diminished sense of smell or taste may suggest the presence of nasal polyps. Common questions include: "What seems to trigger your attack?" "What are your attacks like?" Asthma often worsens at night and the patient may be asked, "Do you ever awaken with an attack?" The timing of attacks other than at night is also important. A relationship between asthma and hormonal influences should be explored. Many women note increased asthmatic symptoms before their period, as well as changes during pregnancy. The physician will ask about the effect of exercise on the patient's symptoms since asthma may occasionally occur only with exercise. Emotional factors will also be investigated as potential triggers: "Are you under more stress?"

A thorough family history will be obtained since the presence of asthma or allergy in closely related family members will support the diagnosis. The physician also will ask about occupation and possible exposures to irritating chemicals, dust, or fumes. To help establish the hyperresponsiveness evident in asthma, the physician will ask how the patient reacts to changes in temperature, humidity, or air pollution, or to the presence of cigarette smoke, fumes, or odors. Reactions to foods containing sulfites as well as to drugs (especially aspirin and penicillin) are also important historical factors.

Looking for Asthma Triggers. When obtaining the initial history, the physician must be a detective, especially in examining sources of irritation that may have precipitated or irritated an underlying asthmatic condition. Both the home and workplace must be reviewed in that context. Many patients are aware of the "sick building syndrome" in which asthma may be produced by a particular contaminant and thus are able to give important information. The type of heating and cooling systems in place should be known. Although the patient may be a nonsmoker, sources of secondhand smoke should be investigated. Other questions to expect include: "Have you recently moved or renovated?" "Do you have pets?" "How often do you clean your humidifier?" If attacks occur frequently at night the bedroom should be singled out for review. "Do you have a mattress cover?" "What type of bedroom floor covering do you have?"

It is not unusual for a patient to supply information that may identify a specific source of irritation and asthma attacks. A thirty-four-year-old man was referred to me for asthma that was extremely difficult to control. He had had many severe attacks and was receiving several asthma medications. Corticosteroids had been prescribed several times, and he had noted side effects of weight gain and stomach upset. The patient noted that he was often well during the day but worsened at night, especially after returning to his apartment. The patient frequently worked in his bedroom where he spent a great deal of time when he was home. He was often awakened during the night by wheezing and shortness of breath and noted that he was "worse in the morning." Asthma attacks regularly occurred whenever he attempted to clean his apartment. I suspected he was allergic to dust mites and that was confirmed by allergy testing. The patient acquired a mattress cover and began following several recommendations mentioned in Chapter 6. He returned for a visit after six weeks and noted he was now sleeping through the night and waking up without wheezing. His medications were sharply reduced, and he has not required further corticosteroids. I often remind him that the credit for his improvement belongs to his mattress cover.

Participating in Your Care. Patients can be extremely helpful by detailing that type of specific information for the physician. Write down the important facts in your medical history that you want to present to your physician. If this narrative is lengthy, send the material ahead of you with other medical records so your physician can review it in detail before your visit. You can be an active participant in your care. Start at the initial interview with your physician. The more detailed information you can supply, particularly in the areas noted previously, the more accurate the diagnosis will be. It is also helpful to describe to your physician how your symptoms have affected your life at home and at work. It is extremely helpful for your physician to know what kind of support you as a patient can rely on as well as whether there are any adverse influences in your life, either environmental or emotional. Reviewing this material is time-consuming and addressing the relief of asthma may take precedent, so tell your physician you want to discuss certain topics at another time. Use a portion of each office visit to discuss a specific topic.

Too often patients are treated only when severe asthmatic symptoms emerge, often requiring emergency room (ER) care. While this is essential and often lifesaving, the "quick fix" of ER treatment is not designed for the careful historical review needed to make the correct diagnosis of asthma.

The Physical Examination

The next step in the diagnosis of asthma is the physical examination, where your physician seeks to correlate the historical information you have provided. For example, the skin and nasal passages are examined for allergic manifestations such as eczema and rhinitis. In the nose, the finding of nasal polyps identifies the patient as someone who may have severe asthma or allergy.

Examination of the chest is extremely important. The physician will note the quality of the breath sounds as air is inhaled and exhaled. When there is airway obstruction, the flow of air through the bronchial tubes is turbulent and often creates wheezing, which is more commonly noted upon exhaling. In addition, the narrowed passages prolong the time it takes for air to be exhaled and the physician will note a prolonged expiratory phase. Although the patient's breathing may be quiet at rest, when asked to take a deep breath and exhale, wheezing and cough may occur then. This maneuver enables a physician to discover an airway obstruction.

Asthma Without Wheezing ("Cough Asthma")

In the last several years, it has become clear that a group of patients with all the characteristics of asthma (airway obstruction, inflammation, and hyperresponsiveness) may never manifest wheezing. In these patients a persistent cough is the main symptom. Although the physical exam may be unremarkable, these patients often have typical histories of cough attacks at night or triggered by exposure to allergens. Laboratory evaluation usually will demonstrate all the features of asthma. This syndrome is frequently identified as the "asthma equivalent syndrome" or "cough asthma." In the past too much weight has been put on the presence of wheezing in the diagnosis of asthma.

Wheezing Without Asthma

Just as the absence of wheezing has often led to patients being misdiagnosed as nonasthmatic, the presence of wheezing also may lead to the erroneous diagnosis of asthma. It has been said that "all that wheezes is not asthma" since many illnesses may produce turbulent airflow through the airways. Too often patients are "diagnosed" simply on this one physical finding.

Wheezing may occur in a variety of illnesses, such as when lesions produce a fixed blockage or obstruction in an air passage. In a child or an adult this may be as simple as a foreign body that has been aspirated. In these cases wheezing may be localized to one area or one lung, which should alert the physician to such a possibility. The history of onset may have been sudden, following a "choking spell." In an adult with a history of smoking, a lung tumor that may be benign or malignant may also produce wheezing by growing within the bronchial tube and blocking the airflow. In these and similar cases, chest x-rays and diagnostic techniques such as bronchoscopy often produce the correct diagnosis.

Emphysema and Chronic Bronchitis. Many respiratory illnesses are characterized by wheezing and may be mistaken for asthma. Emphysema is a disease in which the elasticity of the lung is reduced, usually resulting in closure of the airways. The term "floppy airways" is often used in this disease to describe how easily the bronchial tubes may close and produce wheezing. Chronic bronchitis is a disease in which there is chronic cough and mucus production. Wheezing usually is produced by the clogged and inflamed airways of these patients.

Cystic Fibrosis and Bronchiectasis. Patients with cystic fibrosis, a genetic deficiency disease occurring in children and young adults, often have wheezing due to abnormally viscous mucus clogging their bronchial tubes. A similar mechanism explains the wheezing found in patients with bronchiectasis, an illness in which infections have permanently damaged the bronchial tubes, leading to plugging and inflammation.

Heart Failure ("Cardiac Asthma"). In patients with heart failure, fluid may collect in the lungs around or within the bronchial tubes. These patients often complain of shortness of breath and wheezing, especially at night, mimicking the asthma patient. Due to these similar features this has been called "cardiac asthma" although it is a heart syndrome that tends to resolve with mobilization of the lung fluid by specific medication. The diagnosis often is made by additional physical findings of heart disease as well as by chest x-ray and other heart function tests.

Laryngeal Asthma. A rare but increasingly reported illness that produces wheezing and may be misdiagnosed as asthma is vocal cord dysfunction syndrome. This syndrome also is known as "laryngeal asthma" since in this illness wheezing is produced at the voice box by an abnormal closure of the vocal cords when the patient breathes in (inspiration). Normally, the vocal cords separate on inspiration allowing more air to flow into the lungs. In these patients the sounds of turbulent flow are transmitted over the lung fields, mimicking the wheezing of asthma. The cause of this disorder is unknown. It is thought to be involuntary and often responds to voice therapy. The diagnosis may only be made by direct visualization of the vocal cords by the physician. This is increasingly done with a fiberoptic scope. Pulmonary function testing (see Chapter 2) may also suggest this diagnosis.

The Next Step

Up to this point the physician has used his interview techniques to obtain an accurate patient history and his physical diagnostic skills to form a working diagnosis of bronchial asthma. In order to confirm that impression, laboratory testing and especially pulmonary function testing will be required. These techniques are discussed in Chapter 2.

2

Laboratory Evaluation
of Asthma

FOLLOWING THE CAREFUL review of the patient's history and physical examination, the physician will proceed to several commonly used laboratory tests to complete the diagnostic evaluation. There is no universal "checklist" of tests for every patient since there is great variation in each case. Physicians may also have differences in their laboratory evaluations. A new test for the diagnosis and management of asthma has been approved but is not yet in widespread use.

Blood Tests

In the laboratory evaluation of asthma, it would be common to evaluate the patient's blood count, looking for "allergy cells" called eosinophils. The physician may also obtain an Immunoglobulin E (IgE) level. IgE is the immunoglobulin in the blood that is often elevated in allergic patients. Further allergy testing also may be done through blood analysis, as discussed later in this chapter.

X-Rays

A chest x-ray is often necessary to exclude many of the entities discussed in Chapter 1 that can mimic asthma. However, it does not serve to confirm the diagnosis since the features of asthma occurring within the bronchial tubes cannot be seen on a chest x-ray.

Occasionally, the chest x-ray may show the lungs are greatly expanded and appear larger than normal, or hyperinflated. This occurs in asthma because air may enter the bronchial tubes but have difficulty being exhaled, also known as "air-trapping." This x-ray finding cannot be used as a diagnostic tool for asthma since the same finding may occur in emphysema and in some cases of bronchitis.

Often the physician will order sinus x-rays as part of the laboratory evaluation. Evidence of sinusitis or nasal polyps would identify patients as high-risk candidates for asthma. In addition, the sinusitis may be viewed as a potential aggravating factor in asthmatic attacks and thus become a focus of treatment of individual patients. There is a recent trend toward using the more detailed CAT scan for this exam because of the increased information it provides.

Sputum Exam

Examination of swabs of nasal mucus or chest phlegm (sputum) may be helpful in diagnosing asthma. Microscopic examination may identify abundant eosinophils that would be characteristic of allergy and asthma. The presence of pus cells called neutrophils would suggest an infectious process such as, for example, bronchitis or sinusitis. The physician may request a culture of the coughed sputum if pus cells are seen under the microscope.

Analysis of Exhaled Air for Nitric Oxide

In 2003 the Food and Drug Administration (FDA) approved the NIOX Nitric Oxide Test System for diagnosing and monitoring asthma. This simple test resembles the breathalyzer test used to measure the amount of alcohol in the blood. It is based on the observation that asthmatics exhale much more nitric oxide than normal people. This is thought to be due to the inflammation in asthmatic airways.

To use the test device, the patient inhales air that is free of nitric oxide through a mouthpiece connected by a tube to a computer and then slowly exhales into the mouthpiece. The computer screen immediately displays the amount (concentration) of nitric oxide in the exhaled air. The test requires only a few seconds and has proved extremely helpful in diagnosing asthma in children who are too young to describe their symptoms.

This test has also proved useful in monitoring patients with asthma. Higher levels of exhaled nitric oxide indicates worsening of the condition, while lower levels indicate a response to medication such as inhaled corticosteroids, which reduce inflammation. Physicians equipped with this device may base adjustments in medications on exhaled nitric oxide levels.

The test system is currently expensive, which has limited its use. The analyzer may also be difficult to maintain, and patients may not yet be reimbursed by insurance companies for this test. Two companies are working on making portable, less expensive machines, which should be available in the next two years.

Pulmonary Function Testing

The most important laboratory test the physician performs in the diagnosis of asthma is pulmonary function testing. Before the testing begins, the patient's age, race, sex, height, and weight are recorded. From these statistics the expected normal values are determined. These are called the predicted normals, and they are determined from statistical analysis of large groups of normal subjects.

Forced Expiratory Maneuver

The most common pulmonary function test involves a device known as a spirometer, which measures the amount of air (volume) expelled by the patient as well as its speed (flow) as the air is exhaled forcefully. In this simple but extremely important maneuver, the patient is asked to take a full, deep breath in, then exhale fully and forcefully—this is called a maximum forced expiratory maneuver. In tracing this maneuver the physician determines the maximum amount of air the patient can expel after the deepest inhalation. This amount is called the vital capacity. Figure 2.1 shows a patient performing pulmonary function testing.

As air is expelled the airflow is measured throughout the maneuver until the patient is unable to exhale further. One extremely useful measurement is of the greatest flow that can be obtained after the patient has inhaled fully and forcefully exhaled. This is called peak expiratory flow rate, or "peak flow." This important and easily performed measurement will be discussed in Chapter 3. Flow rates are recorded at the beginning, middle, and end of the forced exhalation maneuver and so is the amount of air expelled each second. As air is exhaled by the lungs, the large bronchial tubes (large airways) empty first with the smaller passages (small airways) contributing a greater share as exhalation continues and ends. In one

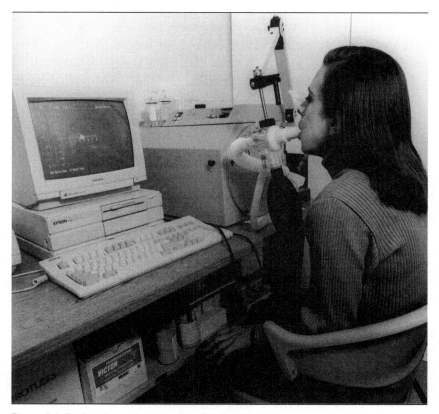

Figure 2.1 Performing pulmonary function tests

second a certain amount of air should normally be exhaled with an expected increase as time increases. The one-second measurement is often a good reflector of the large airways, and measurements toward the middle and end of the breath usually determine the condition of smaller air passages.

Evaluating the Effect of Asthma Medication

Since asthma has been defined as an illness characterized in part by airway obstruction, it is essential for diagnosis to demonstrate this by using spirometry. The definition also includes the feature of reversibility, which means airflow can improve significantly. To demonstrate this feature, spirometry is performed before and after inhaling bronchodilator medication. To be significant, the physician looks for at least a 15 percent improvement in the spirometry parameters after the patient inhales bronchodilator medication.

Diseases such as emphysema, chronic bronchitis, cystic fibrosis, or bronchiectasis may demonstrate severe degrees of airflow obstruction without any improvement after bronchodilator use. However, it may be difficult to demonstrate reversibility in all asthmatics during a single laboratory session, possibly due to severe degrees of bronchial narrowing or inadequate inhalation of medication by the patient. Therefore, the absence of reversibility should never be taken as absolute proof that asthma is not present.

Further Testing

Besides simple spirometry, the physician may perform other pulmonary function tests to better assess and define a patient's condition. Patients with a variety of illnesses may have reduced capacities and flow rates and further testing may be needed. These tests include measurement of lung volume in which the different divisions, or "compartments," of the lungs are measured. These divisions represent quantities of air that are distributed throughout the lung. One example would be the quantity of air that remains in the lung at all times to keep it expanded.

Measuring lung volumes may be performed by two methods. A common technique requires inhaling a special gas mixture containing helium that the patient breathes for several minutes. Analyzing the amount of helium exhaled allows the physician to calculate how the air was distributed in the different air divisions of the lung. Another technique for measuring lung volumes requires an airtight box called a body plethysmograph. In this technique the patient sits in a clear box that resembles a phone booth and breathes against a mouthpiece. By analyzing pressure changes in the box as the patient breathes, it is possible to determine the volume of gas in the lungs.

Another important pulmonary function test is known as a diffusion capacity. This is a sensitive test for the loss of gas exchanging units of the lung as in emphysema. These units are the air sacs or alveoli described in Chapter 1. In this test the patient again breathes a special gas mixture and an amount of exhaled gas is collected. By determining how fast the inhaled gas has disappeared, it is possible to determine whether the air sacs are exchanging gases normally.

Exercise Testing

The tests just described are performed with the patient at rest. Since exercise may create narrowing of the airways, an exercise test may be extremely helpful in demonstrating that a patient develops asthma with exercise or that a patient with mild disease has worse airflow parameters after exercise. Such a test may be performed with a treadmill or a stationary bicycle. The patient is asked to slowly increase the level of exercise until either a certain heart rate is achieved or shortness of breath develops. At this point the patient is asked to perform spirometry and the airflows are compared to those obtained prior to exercise. If the exercise produces significant narrowing of the air tubes, the flow rates will be lower, confirming an asthmatic response. This procedure usually requires less than ten minutes of exercise and is performed under close observation.

Bronchial Challenge Testing

A challenge test may be used by the physician to demonstrate that a patient with a normal result on pulmonary function testing may indeed have asthma. This bronchial challenge or provocation testing would only be performed if the patient's history and physical findings suggested that the patient is asthmatic but spirometry was normal. It is not a routine part of pulmonary function testing. The substances or agents commonly used for challenge testing include histamine, methacholine, and cold air.

Histamine is stored in allergy cells such as mast cells and is released during allergic or asthmatic attacks. It is thought to be one of the mediators of asthma. For this reason it is very suitable for provoking asthma in challenge testing. Methacholine is a chemical that stimulates one part of the nervous system called the parasympathetic nervous system to fire. If inhaled into the bronchial tubes in an asthmatic subject, methacholine will trigger impulses that produce airway constriction. Cold air irritates the bronchial tubes and may also be used for challenge testing. In an asthmatic subject with hyperreactive airways, inhaling cold air will produce significant tightening of the bronchial tubes.

In the patient thought to have occupational asthma, the specific offending substance may be used to confirm the direct link between the substance and the patient's asthmatic reaction. A similar challenge test has been used in patients to confirm allergy to sulfites and aspirin. With any challenge test there is a risk of a severe asthmatic reaction, and for this reason these tests are reserved for difficult diagnostic situations and are only performed under careful observation and control.

Guidelines have been developed for performing and interpreting bronchial challenge testing. It is vital to standardize this type of testing to avoid "false positive" or "false negative" results. Generally, for a provocation test to be positive there must be at least a 15 percent fall in airflow after inhaling the challenge material.

Testing Oxygen Levels

Assessing enrichment of the blood with oxygen by the lung can be made by a noninvasive technique called oximetry, in which a sensor placed on the fingertip or earlobe can accurately measure oxygen saturation. Such a sensor is often immediately placed on an asthmatic patient who has been admitted to an emergency room.

Oxygen saturation testing measures how much oxygen the blood has acquired in the air sacs of the lungs.

The oximeter transmits different wavelengths of light through small blood vessels called capillaries. The fingernail and earlobe are used since these small vessels are close to the surface of the skin. In these small blood vessels, oxygen is carried by a protein called hemoglobin. As oxygen is used by the body, the hemoglobin undergoes a change that can be detected by a different absorption of light from the oximeter. This determination is made during each pulse beat and from the relative amounts of hemoglobin with and without oxygen, the saturation is determined. The patient's pulse is also recorded. Figure 2.2 shows the pulse oximeter in use.

This technique can be extremely helpful in evaluating bronchial asthma since oxygen levels will typically fall with significant degrees of airway obstruction. An asthma attack that reduces oxygen levels signifies a more severe episode and calls for aggressive medical treatment. Oximetry is painless and does not require blood sampling.

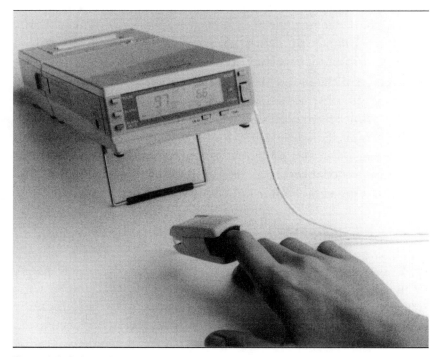

Figure 2.2 Pulse oximeter

Arterial Blood Gases. A more accurate and revealing, although more invasive, test of gas exchange by the lung is called an arterial blood gas. In this test, blood is obtained from an artery (commonly the radial artery at the wrist), allowing a more accurate test of not only the oxygen level but carbon dioxide. Carbon dioxide (CO_2) is the waste product of the body excreted by the lungs. Severe degrees of lung disease, including asthma, can impair gas exchange mechanisms to the point that levels of CO_2 will rise. In bronchial asthma this finding identifies an extremely severe and serious attack that requires hospitalization. These patients will also have lowered oxygen levels and may require mechanical respiratory assistance.

Allergy Evaluation: Is It Necessary?

As a rule, all patients with bronchial asthma should have an allergy evaluation. In children, allergy clearly plays a significant role in the severity of the disease and the frequency of attacks. In adults, the role of allergy is less important although the majority of patients, when tested, are found to be allergic.

Allergy Skin Tests

Although useful as a screening test, the IgE level by itself is not sufficient to determine the presence of allergy (also called atopy). Additional evaluation may include allergy skin testing for specific substances known as allergens that may trigger asthma attacks. This method has been used for more than 100 years and represents an extremely reliable way of determining the presence of allergy to a specific substance. Skin testing is performed by pricking, scratching, or injecting the skin with a small amount of allergen. Positive reactions, which resemble hives, are noted in twenty to thirty minutes. But skin testing is time-consuming and may cause total body reactions in highly sensitive individuals.

Allergy Blood Tests

Evidence for allergy may also be obtained through blood testing that detects the presence of specific antibodies to various allergens.

One technique is the radioallergosorbent test (RAST). This test utilizes radioactive material and detects the presence of a specific IgE antibody that has been produced against a certain allergen. Multiple allergens may be assessed through one sample, which may be particularly helpful in young children. This method, however, is thought to be less accurate than skin testing, although it may prove useful in selected individuals. Other drawbacks include greater cost when compared to skin testing as well as a delay of up to several days in obtaining results.

Allergic Reaction

A positive allergy test does not always identify a significant allergy, so the patient's history becomes an extremely important factor in correlating allergy test results with true triggers of asthma attacks.

Immediate and "Late" Reactions. Allergy reactions are often immediate and severe as in the patient who is allergic to bee venom, but an allergic reaction may not always be immediately apparent. Recently, it has been demonstrated that a "late phase" response may occur several hours after exposure to an offending substance. In the late phase reaction, inflammation plays a significant role and it is essential that effective therapy be directed at this component as well as to bronchial obstruction. If not treated, this late phase reaction may form the basis of recurrent and increasingly severe asthma attacks.

Allergy Treatment: Avoidance and Immunotherapy

Once specific allergens have been identified, the patient must attempt to avoid these substances and clear them from the home and workplace as much as possible. A natural extension of the identification of allergy is the consideration of desensitization or immunotherapy by an allergy specialist. Allergy "shots" are given after sensitivity to specific allergens has been identified. These injections contain extremely small amounts of the allergen, which are slowly increased. These injections produce a "blocking antibody" that interrupts the allergy reaction. Studies of immunotherapy in asthmatics have shown a reduction in symptoms and inhibition of the late asthmatic response. The administration of immunotherapy is a gradual process, often requiring weeks or months to achieve a response. In older subjects the response to treatment may not be as pronounced as in younger patients. Extremely sensitive patients may experience generalized allergic reactions to the administration of allergens.

Recent studies have focused on fatal reactions to allergy injections. The majority of these cases were patients with severe asthma who had histories of severe asthmatic attacks that required steroids and hospitalization. These patients also appeared to be highly sensitive individuals who may have had a previous reaction to allergen injection.

Who Should Be Treated?

In patients with mild or moderate asthma who are well controlled on medication, allergy injections or immunotherapy should not be necessary. Those patients who are unstable should be considered candidates for treatment. In those allergic patients whose symptoms are more severe or who require frequent or continuous administration of corticosteroids, the potential benefits of immunotherapy should be weighed against the potential for severe reactions. Once a response to immunotherapy is obtained, the patient may remain on maintenance therapy for several years.

After the Diagnosis Is Made

After using these laboratory methods to confirm the diagnosis of bronchial asthma, the physician will begin to work closely with the patient to prevent asthmatic attacks. In order for this "working partnership" between physician and patient to be successful, it is necessary to understand the nature of the attack. The asthmatic attack and how to recognize it before it becomes severe are discussed in Chapter 3.

3

The Asthmatic Attack

An asthmatic attack is one of the most striking medical emergencies. One of my first experiences with severe asthma was in the intensive care unit of Bellevue Hospital. I had been called to consult on a fifty-six-year-old woman who was having a severe asthmatic attack. As I entered the unit and approached the bedside, I noted several physicians already in attendance. The patient was sitting upright with labored breathing, and I could hear her wheezing from several feet away. It was clear that she was not doing well despite continuous oxygen and medicated aerosol treatment. Unable to speak due to shortness of breath, her expression was one of fear and desperation. Several days later, greatly improved after vigorous treatment, I asked her to describe what she had been feeling during her attack. "It was like I was drowning."

In the asthmatic attack there is constriction, or tightening, of the bronchial wall muscle and secretion of mucus, often with "plugging" of small air tubes, as well as inflammation and swelling of the bronchial lining. (See Figure 3.1.) The end result is blockage or obstruction of the bronchial tubes. The frequency, duration, and severity of the asthmatic attack vary markedly from patient to patient.

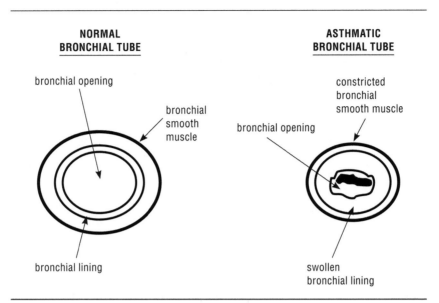

Figure 3.1 Comparison of normal and asthmatic bronchial tubes

Symptoms and Signs of an Attack

Although there are differences from patient to patient, the asthma attack is typically characterized by shortness of breath and wheezing. Cough and mucus production may be prominent symptoms. In some patients wheezing may not occur and a cough may be the dominant symptom. The patient demonstrates a rapid rate of breathing, often with heaving of the chest and use of neck muscles to assist each breath. During an attack the patient is totally disabled. Even speech may be impossible due to severe breathlessness. The patient may be totally consumed by the effort to breathe and unable to eat or dress. The patient is often restless and unable to lie flat. Severe attacks may end in exhaustion, with ominous slowing of the respiratory rate and arrest of breathing.

Depending on the severity of the patient's disease, the attack may be totally or partially reversible, allowing the patient to assume normal activities between episodes. Patients with severe asthma, however, may remain to some degree symptomatic at all times.

It should be noted that the degree of wheezing can be misleading. The severity of the asthmatic attack should never be judged on this basis alone. Some patients who are capable of moving large amounts of air may produce more turbulence and audible wheezing than others who are so severely obstructed that their breaths are shallow and incapable of producing much sound.

How to Recognize the Asthmatic Attack: The Peak Flow Meter

In bronchial asthma it is extremely important to recognize the presence of an attack before it becomes severe and requires emergency measures. Each patient should have a means of assessing the degree of asthma that is present from day to day. In this manner severe episodes and often the use of oral or injectable corticosteroids necessary for such emergencies can be avoided. As an extension of this home monitoring, the patient should be instructed how to respond to the presence of increased asthma. In this way a contingency plan can be in place and ready before severe attacks occur and require emergency room care. The cornerstone of this home monitoring is the peak flow meter. In essence it is an "early warning" device for individuals with asthma.

What the Peak Flow Meter Measures

The peak flow meter is a simple and inexpensive device that can be used anywhere to monitor bronchial asthma and similar conditions. This compact device determines the maximal expiratory flow rate that the patient is capable of producing. Similar to the office spirometry, the patient inhales fully and then exhales fully and forcefully into the flow meter device. A simple scale registers the peak flow. If done as instructed, this flow rate correlates well with other measurement of airflow through the large airways of the lung. With a diary to record readings, the patient can maintain an accurate assessment of the degree of asthma from day to day. This is not unlike the diabetic who records blood sugar readings. Two peak flow meters are shown in Figure 3.2.

Peak flow measurements can be invaluable to the physician in managing patients with bronchial asthma since it gives an objective measurement to go by instead of trying to assess asthma by the degree of shortness of breath or wheezing. Communication with

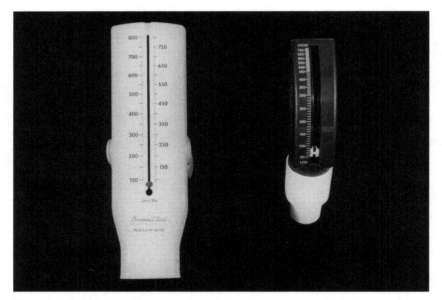

Figure 3.2 Peak flow meters

the physician can be much more meaningful with a record of the patient's peak flows, resulting in earlier and better treatment. With earlier recognition of an attack through peak flow measurements, severe and potentially fatal asthma attacks may be avoided.

Electronic peak flow meters are now available in several forms. Two examples are AirWatch and Piko-1. These more sophisticated and expensive devices (about twice the cost of the mechanical flow meters) are capable of storing several hundred peak flow measurements. Patients may also download their readings by phone to a central computer, which then faxes the results to the physician.

Asthma with Normal Peak Flows

Remember that peak flow measurements reflect primarily large airways and, therefore, do not totally assess the asthmatic condition. Normal peak flows may occur in the presence of significant small airway disease that requires continued and effective treatment. This explains why patients may continue to be symptomatic even with normal peak flow rates.

How Do I Perform a Peak Flow Measurement?

It is extremely important that peak flows be obtained in the same manner each time so that they can be compared. The meter itself should first be inspected to see that the scale indicator has been returned to zero. The patient should sit or stand with good posture, inhale as deeply as possible (maximal inspiration), and then place the meter in the mouth with lips closed around it and exhale fully and forcefully (maximal expiration). A scale records the result. I suggest performing the maneuver three times and recording the best result. Figure 3.3 shows a patient correctly performing the peak flow measurement. Figure 3.4 is an example of a peak flow diary in which readings are recorded.

Obtaining Your Personal Best Value

Once the patient has obtained and begun to use a peak flow meter, it is helpful to record his or her "personal best effort." This result

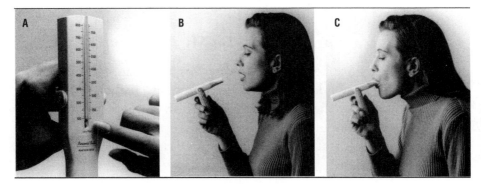

Figure 3.3 Performing peak flow measurement
A. First, set meter to zero.
B. Take a deep breath in.
C. Then blow out as hard as you can!

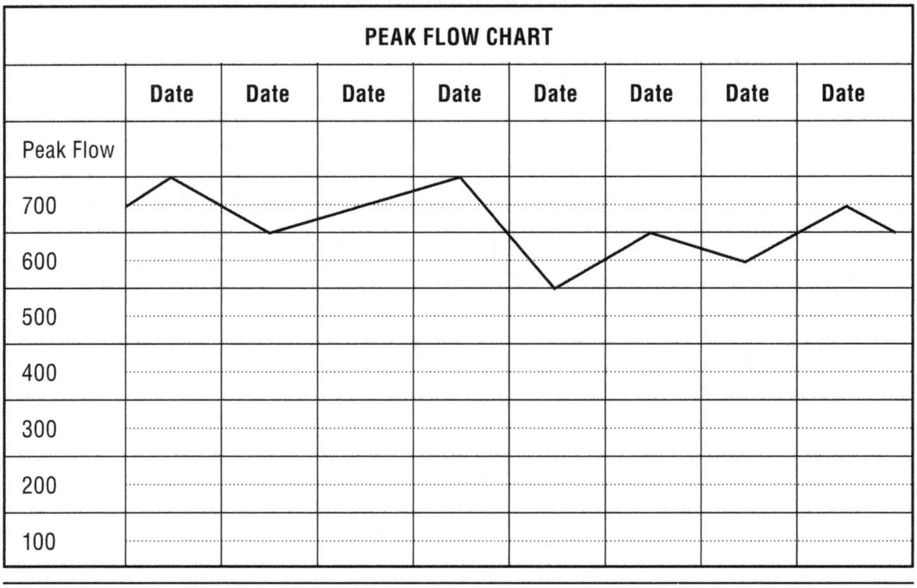

PEAK FLOW CHART								
	Date	Date	Date	Date	Date	Date	Date	Date
Peak Flow								
700								
600								
500								
400								
300								
200								
100								

Figure 3.4 Sample of a peak flow diary

can be used as a reference value to determine if the patient's asthma is stable, improving, or deteriorating.

When Should I Do My Peak Flow?

Peak flows are best if they are performed at approximately the same time each day, preferably morning and night, since asthma may worsen at night. When the peak flow meter is first obtained, the patient may gain useful information by performing flow before and after medication to determine how this influences his or her "personal best."

Using Peak Flows for Diagnosis

Peak flows may also have diagnostic value. Patients may be helped by determining the change in flow in different environmental settings. For example, those who often develop symptoms at work may perform flows at home and work and find that the change in environment produces decreased flows. Investigation of the offending environment may reveal the presence of allergens or pollutants that can be eliminated. Consistently lower flow in a patient's bedroom may suggest that dust mites are in great concentration. A simple remedy may be pillow and mattress covers.

Another diagnostic test that patients may perform is determining peak flows before and after exercise. Although a formal exercise test performed in the physician's office is usually needed to diagnose exercise-induced asthma (EIA), or to demonstrate that patients with established asthma may worsen with exercise, the patient can often gain useful information with the small, portable peak flow meter.

How Should I Interpret Changes in My Peak Flow?

The greatest value of the peak flow meter is as an "early warning" system for the patient's bronchial asthma. It is important to first establish your normal or "personal best" value. From large numbers of volunteers predicted normal values are available for reference. It should be noted that the patient's normal may not equal what is predicted, and it is best to use peak flow results in reference to the patient's best result. Flow is expressed as liters per minute (L/min).

Using the Reference Value

If your best peak flow has been 300 L/min, this should be the reference value you would consider your "normal" result. This may increase with treatment and, therefore, the higher value will become the reference value. Peak flows vary with sex, age, and body size. Remember that peak flow will vary with effort. If a less than maximal effort is given, then falsely low readings will be obtained. This is why the patient should always try to perform the peak flow measurement in the same way and why three efforts should be performed each time.

Interpreting Drops in Peak Flow

When asthmatic attacks occur, peak flows drop due to constriction of the airways. For the patient with a personal best of 400 L/min, a drop of 50 percent to 200 L/min indicates a severe attack and the need for aggressive treatment. The value of the peak flow meter is also its ability to detect less severe drops in flow that allow the patient to administer treatment as outlined by the physician. Therefore, a decrease of 25 percent to 300 L/min identifies a mild to moderate attack. If appropriate treatment is given at this time, then a severe attack may be avoided. Treatment at this point may not include the use of corticosteroids, whereas more severe attacks will commonly require steroid use.

When Your Peak Flow Is Normal

Peak flow measurements may be helpful in a positive way. Shortness of breath may occur from a variety of sources, including anxiety. Patients with severe breathlessness who obtain normal peak flows may benefit greatly from this positive reinforcement and may then focus on other possible sources of this symptom other than asthma.

Who Should Use a Peak Flow Meter?

Any asthmatic may benefit from the use of a peak flow meter, but it is most helpful in patients with moderate to severe asthma. Although a peak flow meter is extremely inexpensive and requires only a few seconds to use, peak flows are often not done. A forty-six-year-old patient who has frequent asthmatic attacks often calls for instructions during a severe episode. I can usually hear wheezing over the phone and recognize from her speech pattern that she is short of breath. When I ask for her record of peak flows, she states, "I haven't been doing it lately, but I'll try to do one now." She registers 100 L/min and is instructed to proceed to the nearest emergency room. This typically results in the use of corticosteroids, which may have been avoided if the attack had been recognized earlier.

Unfortunately, this conversation is repeated several times a week with patients who have had severe asthmatic attacks. In many individuals the failure to use a peak flow meter despite severe asthma is one indicator of who may suffer a fatal attack. In my experience these patients often do not take their medications as directed. Frequently, this behavior appears to result from denial. Many patients do not accept that they have asthma and that it is a chronic disease that requires regular monitoring and medication. Only through patient education and counseling can denial be overcome.

A sixty-year-old man with asthma had just finished providing me with his medical history. "I also want you to know that I have a lovely wife and grandchildren and that your job is to keep me alive so I can enjoy them! What can I do to help myself?" A long conversation followed, but I can assure you that it included the use of a peak flow meter.

Having a Treatment Plan

The drop in peak flow to 50 percent of the patient's best identifies a serious attack. The patient should repeat the maneuver to determine if it is reproducible. Each patient should have a plan of treatment that has been worked out with the physician. This will typically call for immediate use of rapidly acting bronchodilator medication delivered as an aerosol. The plan should contain instructions on the use of corticosteroids and notification of the patient's physician. It should be remembered that a treatment plan must be individualized for each patient. An example of a treatment plan is shown in Figure 3.5.

The physician's knowledge of the patient's history will prove invaluable at this time. Patients who have required hospitalization and especially those who have required respirator support for treatment of asthmatic attacks in the past will be advised not to delay treatment decisions. This patient group may require emergency room treatment as will patients with severe attacks who do not rapidly increase their peak flows with bronchodilator medication administered as directed (and not overused).

Francis V. Adams, M.D.

Pulmonary Medicine

Treatment Program for:

Jane Doe

Treatment

Peak Flow Meter: Record your peak flow twice a day. Perform 3 efforts and take the best one. Your predicted normal is 400 L/min.

Asthma Treatment Plan: If your peak flow drops to 300 L/min: increase your bronchodilator spray to every 6 hours on a regular basis. Increase your steroid spray by doubling the number of sprays per day. If you have been using 4 puffs twice a day, increase to 8 puffs twice a day. If your peak flow decreases to 200 L/min: adjust the bronchodilator spray to every 6 hours and start Prednisone at 40 mg a day. Speak to me as soon as possible. If your peak flow decreases to 100 L/min: use your bronchodilator spray immediately; start Prednisone 40 mg and go to the nearest emergency room. Inform this office as soon as possible.

Please call if you have any questions regarding this treatment plan.

Figure 3.5　Sample of written treatment plan for a specific patient

With bronchial asthma it is necessary to be aggressive early in treatment of severe attacks, including the possible use of an emergency room. With early recognition of a severe attack and aggressive treatment at its onset, fatal or near-fatal episodes can be avoided. In the patient group with severe attacks who respond promptly to treatment, the patient's treatment plan may often be continued in the home. With severe attacks this will most certainly require corticosteroids. Communication with the physician is essential and will be more accurate with serial peak flow measurements. Increasing airflows will confirm the effectiveness of treatment and can be used to adjust medication dosage and frequency of administration.

Following a severe attack that has been successfully treated, it is important for the physician and patient to reassess maintenance medication and the treatment plan. The diary of peak flows will be extremely helpful since it may identify a downward trend that began before a severe attack was recognized. Emphasis on earlier recognition may prove helpful in avoiding future attacks.

With each significant attack the physician will look for a "trigger" mechanism that might be prevented in the future. An example would be raking moldy leaves or dusting without a face mask. Avoiding allergens will be stressed in sensitive patients who suffer serious attacks when exposed to these substances. Often the trigger for an asthmatic attack is the common cold. Although this infection cannot be prevented, the patient should be alerted to the possible adverse effects that might result and be prepared to institute the treatment plan.

In many instances the trigger for a severe asthmatic attack cannot be identified. If attacks are frequent, a review of the medical evaluation should be made. Additional allergy tests may be indicated and another careful examination of the home and work environment made. The patient's administration of medication should also be examined and the maintenance medication program reviewed.

What If Avoidance Doesn't Work?

Despite measures to avoid asthma triggers, the patient may still experience asthmatic attacks. These attacks may be frequent and severe and at times require hospitalization. In a small number of patients, these attacks may prove fatal. In Chapter 4, the asthma medications included in a treatment plan are discussed.

4

The Asthma Medications

AN ASTHMA TREATMENT plan will include medication that the physician prescribes after the diagnosis has been made. In this chapter the different types of asthma medications and the methods for administering them will be discussed.

Asthma medication may be roughly divided into two groups. The first group includes medications that reverse the tightness or constriction in the bronchial tubes. These medications are called bronchodilators. They may be short- or long-acting. The second group of medications is aimed at preventing future attacks. These medications are often called anti-inflammatory since they reverse the red, swollen appearance of the inside of the bronchial tubes. The anti-inflammatory medications are *not* used to treat a sudden asthmatic attack.

Bronchodilator Drugs: Beta-Agonists

Since asthma is characterized by narrowing of bronchial tubes caused by tightening of bronchial wall muscle, treatment has traditionally focused on reversing this process, which is called bronchodilation. The medications that produce this effect are bronchodilators. At this time the most effective bronchodilators are the β_2-adrenergic agonists. These drugs are all derivatives of epinephrine, which has effects on both the heart (termed "beta-1") and lung ("beta-2"). Epinephrine is an important hormone produced in the body by the adrenal gland but has been synthesized in the laboratory. The β_2-adrenergic agonists have been developed to be "selective" stimulants of lung structures, with reduced unwanted effects on the heart and blood vessels such as high blood pressure, nervousness, tremors, and palpitations. Their effects are produced through nerve endings called receptors located within the lungs. One such β_2-receptor is located in the muscle layer that surrounds the bronchial tube. With the administration of these agents and stimulation of the receptor, the bronchial wall muscle relaxes, producing bronchodilatation.

Genetics Plays a Role

Recent research into the genetic basis of asthma has revealed that certain individuals are more likely to respond to β_2-adrenergic agonists. In the future DNA analysis may guide β_2-agonist treatment.

Are These Drugs Safe?

This potent and effective group of medications has been the subject of much debate. In the past these agents were often regarded as the only medication necessary for the treatment of asthma. Research has shown that the β_2-adrenergic agonists do not have anti-inflammatory effects nor do they affect bronchial hyperresponsiveness. In view of these facts it has become increasingly clear that they cannot be relied on for the entire treatment of more than mild, intermittent asthma.

It is also clear that despite their extreme effectiveness as bronchodilators, their overuse may be a problem. Unfortunately, overuse of the β_2-agonists is extremely common. Statistics have shown a connection with overuse of one of the short-acting β-adrenergic agonists, fenoterol (Berotec), and fatal asthma. It is not completely clear, however, whether this connection is due to a direct effect of overadministration of this drug or whether it is simply due to the fact that a more severe group of asthmatics were using it. Several researchers have argued that these severe patients may suffer fatal attacks whether they overuse these agents or not.

Controversy also has occurred with the use of long-acting β_2-agonists due to results of studies demonstrating an increased number of asthma deaths among patients using these medications. The question as to whether these medications had a direct cause in these deaths will be addressed under specific medications.

Because of the rapid effect of alleviating asthma (called "rescue") that is achieved by the short-acting β-agonists, patients tend to favor this group of medications over the slower-acting asthma drugs. It is not unusual to find that an asthmatic has stopped using other medications because "they didn't work like my other spray." In this way, patients will often fall into a pattern of overusing this group of medications. It should be stressed that the use of the short-acting β_2-agonists should be on an "as needed" basis whenever possible. This alone identifies a patient who is under good control and has mild asthma. It should also be stressed that other asthma medications can be just as effective in controlling asthma if used properly.

Another area of controversy concerning the β_2-adrenergic agonists is that they are "too effective" and permit patients to expose themselves to unwanted and potentially harmful irritants. A twenty-eight-year-old woman with asthma and severe allergy to cat dander has been under my care for several years. On several office visits for flare-ups of her asthma she mentioned she had recently visited the homes of friends who had cats because she "knew my spray would help me." In fact, she described many visits that ended with her making a "quick exit" even with the use of her β_2-agonist. Each visit would result in overuse of her spray. After discussing the dangers of overuse and the fact that the "late phase" of her attacks might explain why she was not doing well for days after her visits, the patient no longer places herself at unnecessary risk. Unfortunately, many patients continue to do so.

Long-Term Effects of B$_2$-Agonists. One of the most frequent questions that I am asked is whether there are any long-term effects of this group of medications. There is some evidence that use of β-adrenergic agonists may result in an increase in bronchial irritability when they are stopped, producing more asthma. This phenomenon does not appear to be significant when these agents are used as prescribed but may occur with overuse. If increased irritability does occur, it does not appear to be prolonged.

Another common question is whether the effect of the β_2-agonist "wears off" over time. This concern may lead to underuse of an important asthma medication. The great majority of studies of long-term use have not demonstrated that these agents lose their effectiveness. This phenomenon should not occur if the daily dosage is within the limits the physician prescribes but has been seen with overuse. It should be emphasized that the β-adrenergic agonists are safe and effective bronchodilators in the majority of patients when used as directed by the physician. Both of the adverse effects just noted result from patients exceeding the prescribed dosage.

Specific Drugs

The β-agonists were developed in the 1940s, with isoproterenol (Isuprel) the first of the class. Like epinephrine (adrenaline) this agent has both beta-1 and beta-2 effects. Isoetharine (Bronchosol) was one of the first "selective" β_2-adrenergic agonists introduced in the United States, and it was followed by metaproterenol (Alupent). Although designated as "selective," these medications have retained to a reduced extent the property of the parent compound, epinephrine, that produces rapid heartbeat, nervousness, and tremors. These side effects may be particularly disturbing in susceptible individuals, the elderly, and those with underlying heart disease.

With the development of selective β_2-adrenergic agonists there is no place for the use of nonselective agents that have greater stimulatory effects on the heart and circulation. Further research has produced more potent, longer-acting, and more selective agents. Table 4.1 lists the β_2-agonists by generic and brand name as well as the types of preparations that are available.

For the Acute Asthmatic Attack: Short-Acting Agents. Several selective β_2-adrenergic agonists are available for use. These agents are available as aerosol sprays delivered by metered-dose inhalers (MDIs), aerosol solution to be delivered by nebulization, dry

Table 4.1   The B-Adrenergic Agonists

Drug Name	Brand Name	Preparations	Comments
Albuterol	Proventil HFA Ventolin HFA	MDI, tablet, nebulizer, syrup	Selective, short to medium duration DPI available in Europe Generic available with CFC or HFA
Levalbuterol	Xopenex Xopenex HFA	nebulizer MDI	Selective, short to medium duration May have reduced adverse effects
Fenoterol	Berotec	MDI	Selective, short duration, not available in United States
Metaproterenol	Alupent	MDI, nebulizer, tablet, syrup	Less selective, short-acting
Pirbuterol	Maxair	Autohaler	Selective, short to medium duration
Terbutaline	Brethine	injection, tablets	Selective, short to medium duration DPI available in Europe
Salmeterol	Serevent Serevent Diskus	MDI DPI	Long-acting MDI not available in United States
Formoterol	Foradil	DPI	Long-acting; faster onset of action than salmeterol

powders for inhalation (DPI), short- and long-acting tablets, and syrups flavored for children. In the acute asthmatic attack, the treatment of choice for prompt relief of symptoms is the administration of a short-acting β_2-adrenergic agonist. B_2-adrenergic agonists albuterol (Proventil, Ventolin), levalbuterol (Xopenex), metaproterenol (Alupent), pirbuterol (Maxair), terbutaline (Brethine), fenoterol (Berotec), and bitolterol (Tornalate) have a rapid onset of action (within minutes) with duration of action of four to six hours. The recommended dosage is two puffs every four to six hours as needed.

These medications differ in selectivity and potency as well as how fast they begin to work and when their peak effect is reached. There are also differences in how long the effect of the drug lasts. Fenoterol (Berotec) has never been made available in the United States. Its extremely rapid onset of action may have contributed to its overuse, and it has been implicated in cases of fatal asthma in New Zealand.

Levalbuterol. Levalbuterol (Xopenex) is the most recent addition to the family of short-acting β_2-agonists. Man-made ("racemic") albuterol is made up of two parts or isomers, known as "R" and "S." The R-isomer interacts with the β_2-receptor and is responsible for both the benefits (bronchodilatation) and potential side effects (rapid heartbeat, tremors) of this drug. The S-isomer does not interact with the β_2-receptor. It is suspected of having other adverse effects on the clearance of mucus and may possibly promote inflammation. In developing levalbuterol, researchers were able to separate albuterol into these two parts and to eliminate the S-isomer. Initially introduced in liquid form for nebulizer use (two dosage strengths, 0.63 mg and 1.25 mg), levalbuterol has recently been released in a metered-dose spray form (Xopenex HFA). Like albuterol, levalbuterol has a rapid onset of action and can be used every four to six hours. It is designed for "rescue" and should be used only on an "as-needed" basis. Levalbuterol has been approved for children four years of age or older.

Only a few studies have compared levalbuterol to albuterol. In these trials, the 1.25 mg nebulizer solution of levalbuterol appeared to be more potent than the unit dose of albuterol. Further studies are needed to determine whether levalbuterol has significant advantages over albuterol.

Long-Acting B$_2$-Agonists. Longer-acting β_2-adrenergic agonists—salmeterol (Serevent) and formoterol (Foradil)—delivered by metered-dose or dry powder inhaler with a duration of action of up to twelve hours were developed to reduce the frequent use of short-acting agents. These agents provide sustained dilatation of the bronchial tubes and improve asthma control.

Controversy regarding the use of long-acting β-adrenergic agonists began after these agents were introduced outside of the United States. In July 2005 the Food and Drug Administration (FDA) issued a public health advisory alerting "health care professionals and patients that these medicines may increase the chance of severe asthma episodes, and death when those episodes occur." Unfortunately, the results of the studies that led to this advisory are considered indefinite and contradictory evidence has been presented by the manufacturers. Where increased deaths have occurred in relation to either short- or long-acting β_2-agonists, the events have not occurred equally throughout the exposed populations. Patients using inhaled corticosteroids in the studies under question did not have an increased risk of death or asthma exacerbations. These results suggest that the adverse outcomes noted by the FDA were not a direct toxic effect of the drugs but may have been due to the severity of the individual's asthma and a delay in seeking medical care. At this time physicians must weigh the beneficial effects of these long-acting agents on asthma control with their possible rare potential for contributing to severe illness or death.

Salmeterol. Salmeterol is available in the United States alone (Serevent Diskus) or in combination with an inhaled corticosteroid (Advair Diskus) in multidose DPI form. The recommended dosage is two puffs (MDI) or one inhalation (DPI) every twelve hours administered on a regular basis. When compared to albuterol, salmeterol is more potent and more selective. Studies that have compared these two agents have documented that the salmeterol-treated patients have more sustained improvement in their lung function and fewer flare-ups of their asthma. In these studies the salmeterol patients also had fewer nocturnal attacks and awoke with better peak flows.

Formoterol. Formoterol (Foradil) is available in the United States in a single dose DPI form and is administered every twelve hours. It has a faster onset of action than salmeterol (fifteen minutes) with sustained effect up to twelve hours. Formoterol has also been demonstrated to be many times more potent than albuterol with longer lasting improvement in lung function. A combination of formoterol and an inhaled corticosteroid (see Chapter 13) should be available in the United States in 2007.

How Should Long-Acting β_2-Agonists Be Used? The longer-acting β_2-agonists appear to provide patients with more sustained control over their asthmatic symptoms, particularly patients with frequent nocturnal attacks. Salmeterol has also been demonstrated to allow patients who are maintained on topical corticosteroid sprays to reduce their steroid dosages. In addition, the twice-a-day administration provides greater convenience for the patient. It must be emphasized that due to the slower onset of action of the long-acting β_2-agonists these agents must not be used for relief of an acute asthmatic attack. The long-acting β_2-agonists should only be used for maintenance therapy and do not have a role in the treatment of a sudden asthma attack.

Both the short- and long-acting agents administered before exercise are capable of preventing EIA. Salmeterol and formoterol have been compared to albuterol in patients with EIA and appears to have an advantage. The long-acting β_2-agonist-treated patients had more sustained protection against EIA.

How Should the B-Adrenergic Agonist Be Given?

In an acute attack the fastest means of getting this medication to the bronchial tubes is by inhalation. This can be achieved in minutes by inhaling medicated spray administered by a metered-dose inhaler (MDI) or a dry powder inhaler (DPI). A medicated mist generated by a nebulizer can also be used for inhalation.

What Is an Asthma Aerosol?

An asthma aerosol is a mixture of a liquid medication suspended in a gas that can be inhaled. Aerosols differ in the size of the spray or mist particles that are inhaled. Particle size is important since large particles are not likely to reach the bronchial tubes and may land in the mouth or throat. Examples of asthma aerosols are sprays from MDIs and nebulizers. The goal of aerosol therapy is inhalation of active medication with penetration into the bronchial tubes.

Metered-Dose Inhalers

Metered-dose inhalers contain medication in aerosol form. These devices were first introduced in 1956 and have become widely used for asthma and rhinitis. Metered-dose inhalers consist of a canister of medication and an actuator with a mouthpiece. The actuator is the outer shell in which the canister "sits." In the canister, medication is suspended in a mixture of a liquid propellant gas and preservatives. The propellant used in most MDIs has been a mixture of Freon gases called chlorofluorocarbons (CFCs). Due to an ozone-depleting effect on our atmosphere it is being replaced by a non-CFC agent, hydrofluoroalkane (HFA).

When the canister is pressed into the actuator, the mixture of medication and propellant passes through a valve. The release of the contents under pressure transforms the liquid mixture into a spray that can be inhaled. In Figure 4.1 an MDI is diagrammed. Figure 4.2 shows an MDI with a device known as a "spacer" attached.

In the United States, the MDI is the most common means of administering short-acting β-adrenergic agonists. It is a compact and portable device that dispenses a certain amount of medication rapidly. Coordination between hand activation of the MDI and breathing must exist for the medication to be properly delivered. Metered-dose inhalers come in many shapes and sizes. Figure 4.3 shows two commonly used MDIs.

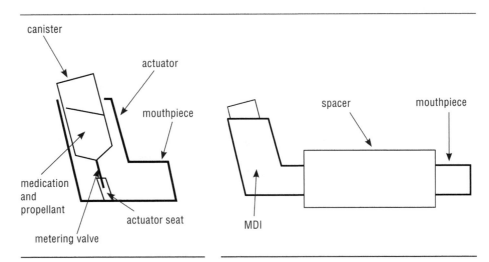

Figure 4.1 Diagram of metered-dose inhaler

Figure 4.2 Diagram of metered-dose inhaler with a spacer

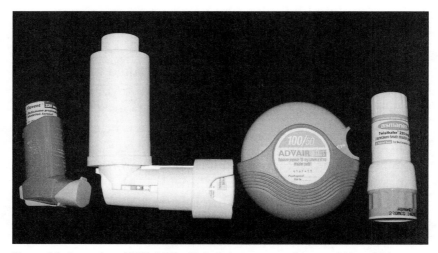

Figure 4.3 Examples of MDI, MDI with built-in spacer, and two multidose DPIs
(l to r)

Although the MDI generally is a safe device, it should be noted that a small number of patients may have adverse reactions to the propellants. This reaction may produce a worsening of asthma symptoms instead of the expected improvement after use of the MDI. Patients also must be careful to keep the mouthpiece of the MDI closed when not in use and free of foreign objects. Many patients have inadvertently aspirated foreign objects such as coins that slipped into the open mouthpiece and were then inhaled. Metered-dose inhalers are frequently kept in a pocket or purse where such foreign objects are usually found, so it is best to carefully check the MDI before using it.

A thirty-two-year-old man under my care for bronchial asthma called me in distress one night stating that "something went wrong when I sprayed." He had been in the habit of keeping his uncovered MDI in his pocket and while shopping had placed loose change in the same pocket. After dinner he had used his MDI and felt "something go in." An x-ray in the emergency room showed a dime lodged in his windpipe. A procedure called bronchoscopy was required to remove it. The patient was released the next day with an MDI that he had carefully capped.

Proper Technique for MDI Use. Proper technique in using an MDI is essential to the effectiveness of the β-adrenergic agonist. It is estimated that only 10 to 14 percent of the medication released reaches the smaller, more peripheral airways of the lung. If the drug is not administered correctly, symptoms will not be relieved, often leading to medication overuse. It is best to practice with a mirror at home after being instructed in the doctor's office.

The preferred method is the closed mouth technique in which the patient closes his or her lips tightly around the mouthpiece. Before activating the spray, shake the inhaler well and "test-fire" the device into the air. You may hold the MDI with both hands if necessary. Before activating the spray, empty your lungs by breathing out fully through the mouth. When you feel the need to inhale, place the mouthpiece completely into the mouth and activate the spray by pressing down on the top of the metal canister. Inhale slowly and deeply over three to five seconds, remove the inhaler from your mouth, and hold your breath, if possible, by counting to five before exhaling again. Do not repeat the second spray in "rapid-fire sequence." Allow at least a minute between sprays. Too often patients will "puff-puff" in a few seconds and then wonder why they have to use their inhalers again "so soon." Proper technique is essential for medication to reach the small airways of the lung. Figure 4.4 shows the proper technique used for the closed mouth method.

Always check the expiration date on the side of the removable metal canister and discard any expired medication. It is best to determine how many puffs are available by the number you have used (keep a record if necessary) or by the date obtained. Mark your calendar when you purchase your inhaler. Most MDIs contain 200 sprays and from your pattern of use it should be easy to calculate how long an MDI will last. A test using a glass of water to determine if the metal canister will float (empty) or sink to the bottom (full) is less accurate than an actual record. Never assume medication is present by the "feel" of the weight of the MDI. Propellants and preservatives are used in MDIs and may give you the false impression that some medication remains.

Common Mistakes. Large studies have documented the difficulty that patients experience with MDIs. It has been estimated

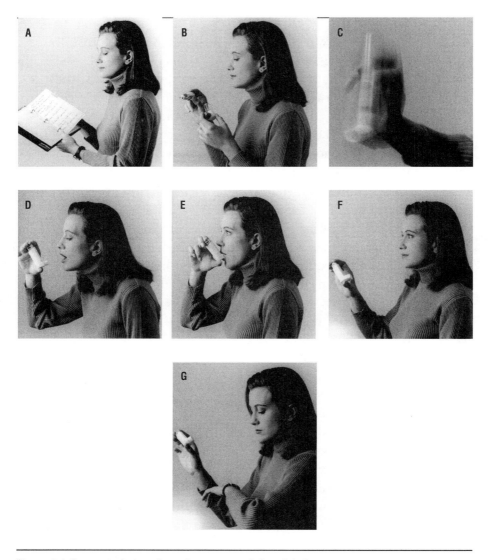

Figure 4.4 Proper technique for using a metered-dose inhaler
A. First, check your calendar for date of purchase.
B. Also check date of expiration on canister.
C. Shake MDI vigorously!
D. Let all the air out of your lungs (exhale).
E. Place mouthpiece in your mouth, close lips around, and depress the top of the canister as you begin a slow, deep, full breath (inhale).
F. Hold your breath for 5–10 seconds (if possible).
G. Exhale and relax: Wait 60 seconds and then repeat steps C–G.

that more than 50 percent of patients use improper technique, with the most common mistake being the "firing" of the medication after inhalation begins, and poor coordination may not improve with repeated instruction. Additional common mistakes include failing to remove the cap and holding the spray upside down. Patients should be encouraged to have the physician observe their technique with the MDI. Videotapes of the proper technique are available and may be obtained from your physician.

About 70 percent of the medication discharged on activation of most MDIs is deposited in the mouth and throat and never reaches the bronchial tubes. Approximately 15 percent remains in the mouthpiece of the MDI and 10 to 15 percent actually reaches the bronchial airways. Ultrafine sprays, such as the inhaled steroid QVAR, that emit smaller particles have been developed with greater delivery of medication into the lungs. Any method that increases deposition of medication into the bronchi is advantageous to the control and treatment of asthma. For treatment to be successful, the coordination between activation of the MDI and inhalation must be fairly precise.

Nebulizers

A nebulizer may also be used to rapidly deliver aerosol medication containing β-adrenergic agonists. This device, which is commonly used in an emergency room setting, is basically a simple system that allows rapidly flowing air or oxygen to be bubbled through a solution containing the drug. This system produces a vapor that the patient inhales. Nebulizers differ in terms of the size of mist particles they produce. It is important to note that the nebulizer does not require the coordination between hand and breathing necessary for MDI use.

Nebulizer delivery of a β_2-agonist is preferred in emergency settings since a greater quantity of the drug can be delivered, approximately four to ten times the amount of medication delivered by two puffs from an MDI. The greater quantity of drug delivered by the nebulizer method may also result in greater side effects (tremors, rapid heartbeat, muscle cramps, nervousness) than those noted after using an MDI. But in an emergency setting the beneficial effect of opening the bronchial tubes usually outweighs any adverse side effects.

Nebulizers may be obtained for the home, but this should not be necessary for most asthma patients. In view of the adverse effects and increased dosage, a home nebulizer should only be prescribed for the most severely afflicted patients with asthma that cannot be controlled with metered-dose sprays or powder. These devices are much more expensive and cumbersome than MDIs, although small portable units are now available. A patient is shown using a nebulizer in Figure 4.5.

Metered-Dose Inhaler Versus Nebulizer Delivery

A number of studies have compared the effectiveness of a β-agonist delivered by an MDI with a spacer attachment and the same drug

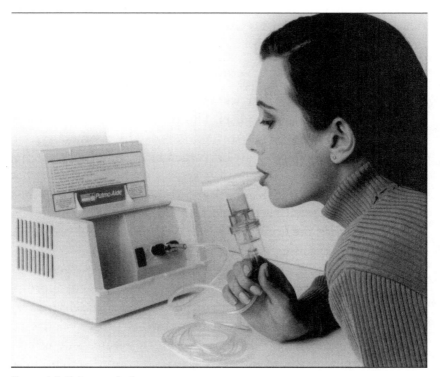

Figure 4.5 Using a nebulizer

delivered by a nebulizer. These studies have shown little or no difference in effectiveness between the two delivery systems. One explanation is that with an MDI the patient takes a deep breath to deliver medication to the bronchial tubes, while with a nebulizer the patient breathes normally. The deep breath may actually be advantageous to the delivery of medication to smaller bronchial tubes. During a severe attack, however, it may be difficult for patients to actively inhale deeply enough. While routine use of a nebulizer for stable asthma should be discouraged, there remains a definite place for nebulizer delivery of medication in patients with severe disease and in an emergency.

Nebulizers also require more maintenance and cleaning than do MDIs. There is a greater risk of contamination with nebulizers and patients must follow a proper cleaning routine.

Breath-Activated Inhaler

In view of the difficulty some patients have coordinating MDIs, great interest has been devoted to the development of a breath-activated inhaler. Pirbuterol (Maxair Autohaler) is available in this form and additional breath-activated devices have been under development. With the Autohaler the patient has to inhale forcefully, activating the mechanism that delivers the dosage of medication. Education in the use of a breath-activated device is also required, but it appears patients achieve mastery of this device faster than with the MDI. In those patients who have good coordination with MDIs, the breath-activated device does not appear to improve delivery of medication. In patients with poor coordination, however, the breath-activated inhaler will improve delivery of bronchodilator medication.

A drawback of the Maxair Autohaler spray is the lack of an override button that would allow the patient to activate the spray if it malfunctions. In addition, patients with severe degrees of narrowing of the bronchial tubes may have difficulty activating the device.

Computer-Driven MDI. A further advancement in breath-activated MDI technology is SmartMist (Aradigm). The handheld, battery-powered device contains a microprocessor that automatically activates MDIs upon correct inhalation. The patient inhales normally through a mouthpiece and is guided by red and green indicator lights to inhale slowly and evenly. Medication is released when the desired flow rate and amount of air inhaled are achieved. Once inhalation is complete, a ten-second timer reminds the patient to hold his breath. This device electronically collects peak flow data that can be transferred to a personal computer and used by the physician. SmartMist has been shown to improve the delivery of aerosol medication and should be of value to patients with moderate to severe asthma.

Respimat Soft Mist Inhaler

Respimat Soft Mist Inhaler is a unique device developed by Boehringer Ingelheim that is propellant-free and delivers a metered dose of medication as a fine mist. The extremely fine mist reduces the deposition of medication in the mouth and throat and increases the amount delivered to the bronchial tubes. The mist moves slowly, which allows the patient to inhale without a forceful inspiration. This device is currently available in Europe; plans for introduction in the United States have not been announced.

Spacers

Patients who experience difficulty with MDIs may benefit from the use of a spacer, or extension tube. Spacers come in different sizes (large or small volume) and shapes. Figure 4.6 shows three spacer devices that are widely used.

The spacer in its simplest form consists of an attachment or holding chamber that fits over the mouthpiece of the MDI. Activation of the inhaler allows the medication to enter the attached chamber, or "spacer," from which the patient then inhales. Use of this device often improves the delivery of medication since it is more difficult for the patient to "lose the medication" by spraying before inhaling. The medication is "trapped" in the spacer for several seconds, allowing the patient to inhale with less fear of "spraying and inhaling at the wrong time."

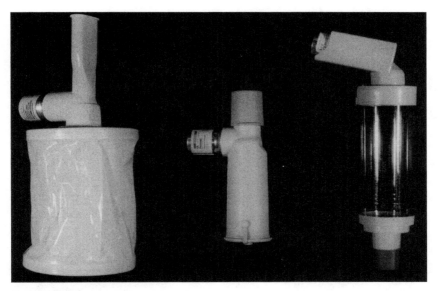

Figure 4.6 Examples of spacers

Studies of various spacers have shown they reduce the amount of medication deposited in the mouth that never reaches the bronchial tubes. Even the simplest device has been shown to reduce by half the amount "lost" in the mouth. Although the amount of medication deposited in the mouth may be reduced by even the simplest spacer, it appears that the larger-volume spacers actually increase the amount of medication that reaches the lungs. Examples of large-volume spacers are InspirEase, InhalAid, and Nebuhaler. InspirEase consists of a collapsible bag and a valve that can signal the patient when inhaling too fast. Aerochamber is a medium-sized spacer with a mouthpiece and one-way valve that can also signal if the patient is inhaling too fast. It is also available with a face mask for small children and adults (Figure 4.7). OptiHaler is an extremely compact spacer that easily incorporates the MDI in its design. Table 4.2 is a partial list of currently used spacers.

Patients with poor technique with an MDI may also experience difficulty with a large-volume spacer. As with the MDI, it is important not to "fire" the medication after the start of a breath. Breathe

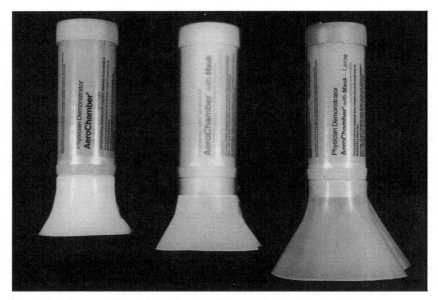

Figure 4.7 Spacer with mask attached in different sizes

in slowly to full inspiration. Some patients have been reluctant to carry around the larger spacers and feel they are cumbersome.

Advantages of a Spacer. Spacers may offer several other advantages with MDIs. The total body absorption of inhaled medication is greatly influenced by the amount deposited in the mouth. This material makes up the highest proportion of medication that is absorbed. By reducing the amount lost in the mouth, spacers reduce total body absorption and may therefore reduce possible total body side effects. With the β-agonists, this may mean reduced nervousness or shakiness after use. This benefit may be advantageous in high doses of inhaled corticosteroids, reducing the chances of steroid side effects on the whole body. Spacers have also been shown to reduce the risk of yeast infection (candidiasis) that may occur with the inhaled corticosteroids.

Another advantage of a large-volume spacer is that in those patients requiring large numbers of puffs of medication, as in high-dose inhaled corticosteroids, the spacer allows the patient to inhale

Table 4.2   Spacer Devices*

Name	Size	Comments
Aerochamber	Medium volume	Rigid, signals fast flow, available with mask for children
InspirEase	Large volume	Collapsible bag, mouthpiece signals if inhaling too fast
Nebuhaler	Large volume	Rigid, mouthpiece
OptiHaler	Small volume	Compact, MDI canister may be carried in device

*This is a partial list of spacer devices and is not intended to be all-inclusive.

two puffs of medication for each inhalation, thus reducing the time the patient must spend inhaling large doses of medication.

Children and Spacers. In children, spacers may be extremely helpful in delivering medication. Children as young as three years of age who would not otherwise be able to use an MDI may benefit from the use of a spacer with a face mask (Aerochamber). Studies of children with asthma that have compared the use of an MDI with a spacer with mask and a nebulizer have found no difference in safety or effectiveness.

Dry Powder Inhalers

β_2-adrenergic agonists as well as inhaled corticosteroids are also available in dry powder form for inhalation. Multidose dispensers are available to assist patients in administering this powder with a minimum of preparation. Single-dose dry powder inhalers (DPI) are also widely available. This form of medication may be particularly helpful with patients who have difficulty with MDIs since with the powder form the patient again performs a breath-activated inhalation after placing the lips tightly around the mouthpiece. In the same maneuver as performed with the MDI, the patient first empties the lungs and then performs a maximal inhalation, thus fully drawing in the powder and then holding the breath.

With environmental concerns growing over the use of CFC propellants that destroy the ozone layer, the use of β-adrenergic agonists and inhaled corticosteroids in powder form will increase. Patient acceptance of this form of medication has been slow, primarily because of unfamiliarity in addition to minor throat discomfort. However, the latter may also occur with the spray form as well as minor changes in voice noted by a few patients.

Patients with arthritis or neurological diseases such as Parkinson's disease may experience difficulty loading the powder capsule into their single-dose DPI. This problem will be eased by use of a multiple-dose powder inhaler. Another possible drawback of powder inhalers is that the amount of medication the patient receives varies with the force of inhalation. Patients who can inhale more forcefully may receive a lot more medication. Another consideration with dry powder inhalers is the potential adverse effect of high temperature and humidity on their function.

Dry powder inhalers are clearly not as versatile as MDIs. Metered-dose inhalers have now been used with patients who are breathing with the assistance of a respirator. The MDI may be fitted with a special adapter that allows medication to be inhaled through the respirator system. For this and other reasons, it is clear that the MDI will remain in widespread use for treatment of bronchial asthma.

Oral Forms of B₂-Agonists

The β-adrenergic agonists available in tablet or elixir form are not for emergency use since they have slow onsets of action (up to one hour). Albuterol, terbutaline, and metaproterenol are available as oral medications. Since they are absorbed into the bloodstream in greater quantity than the inhaled form, there are greater chances of side effects. These include tremors, muscle cramps, nervousness, insomnia, and palpitations. The long-acting oral preparations of albuterol have proved useful for patients with nocturnal asthma, although the long-acting aerosol sprays that have become available also have been effective in this setting. Those patients who have difficulty using an MDI may benefit from the oral preparations.

Another potential advantage of oral preparations is that the medication carried in the blood may reach small bronchial tubes that may not have been reached by inhalation. These small airways are often inflamed and swollen in moderate and severe asthma and receive only a relatively small percentage of the medication inhaled. In addition, there may be thick mucous "plugs" that block the air passages. Aerosol medication, therefore, may be primarily distributed to the larger, more open passages, which receive greater airflow on inhalation. It is conceivable, however, that medication deposited in these larger passages may be absorbed into blood vessels and reach the blood circulation, thereby eventually reaching the smaller airways.

In the asthmatic patient who does not appear to respond fully to aerosol medication, trial with an oral preparation is indicated. Peak flows or spirometry may be performed after a suitable trial of one to two weeks. If flow rates have increased and symptoms have diminished, then the oral preparation of the β_2-adrenergic agonist may be used in conjunction with the aerosol. A drawback to this approach will be the greater likelihood of adverse effects from the increased absorption of the β-agonist. Of note, however, is that tolerance to these effects often develops after several days of use. Unfortunately, the elderly population with asthma may be adversely affected more than younger patients. Tremors may be especially severe in older patients. These patients are also more likely to have preexisting cardiac conditions that may increase the risk of adverse effects such as rapid or irregular heart rhythms.

Should Epinephrine Ever Be Used?

The use of epinephrine by injection for the treatment of asthma dates to as early as 1903. An aerosol form was developed around 1910. For many decades epinephrine was the only available medication for the treatment of bronchial asthma. Its use in the emergency setting has certainly saved countless numbers of lives.

In view of the fact that epinephrine is a nonselective agent that has potent effects on the heart and circulation, its use for treating bronchial asthma has declined. In elderly patients in particular, administration of epinephrine may result in increased blood pressure and heart rate. These effects may contribute to the development of stroke and heart attack. For these reasons, emergency room treatment of bronchial asthma currently consists of the administration of a selective β_2-adrenergic agonist by nebulization.

For Anaphylaxis. Epinephrine is still an important medication for treating severe allergic reactions. It is the treatment of choice for a severe reaction known as anaphylaxis, a total body allergic reaction that may lead to collapse or shock. One example is the severe reaction to a bee sting in a sensitive individual. Injectable preparations of epinephrine (Epipen) that automatically inject a premeasured dose are available by prescription for highly allergic patients.

Over-the-Counter Medication

Over-the-counter nonprescription preparations of aerosol epinephrine (Primatene) should be avoided. These preparations are extremely weak and short-acting. Since their effects may last only a few minutes, they are commonly abused. They also contain CFC propellant, which damages the atmosphere.

With far more effective treatment available for bronchial asthma, I believe these agents should be withdrawn since they may actually deter patients from seeking appropriate and necessary medical attention.

Bronchodilator Drugs: Theophylline

Theophylline has been used for treating bronchial asthma for nearly sixty years, but it is a weaker bronchodilator than the β-adrenergic agonists. Although widely used as a bronchodilator, the mechanism of its action is unclear. The most recent theories suggest an anti-inflammatory effect that is supported by the inhibition of the late phase response. Due to the controversy over its mode of action, theophylline has fallen out of favor and is no longer regarded as a first-line asthma medication comparable to the β_2-adrenergic agonists.

At this time theophylline may still prove useful as a second-line drug. Research has demonstrated that theophylline may allow patients who require high doses of inhaled corticosteroids to reduce their steroid dosages. Patients with intolerance to β-agonist side effects may find they are better able to tolerate theophylline. Its availability as an oral medication in a sustained time-release form may be preferred by some patients. Dosing is usually on a twice-a-day basis, with some patients able to achieve satisfactory results from once-a-day administration. This once-a-day dose is best given in the evening and may prove extremely helpful in treating nocturnal asthma.

Sustained-Release Preparations

Large numbers of sustained-release theophylline preparations are available by prescription, but they may vary in their rate of release of medication into the bloodstream. Once a certain preparation is prescribed, adjustment of the dosage will require follow-up and blood testing. After the proper dosage is established, it is advisable not to substitute one preparation for another since the substitute may not achieve the same results. There is little use for short-acting theophylline preparations since they must be given several times a day.

Intravenous Form: Aminophylline

An intravenous form of theophylline known as aminophylline is available for emergencies. In view of the faster onset of action of the β_2-adrenergic agonists, intravenous aminophylline also is not considered a first-line treatment in an emergency room. Although there is some controversy concerning its effectiveness in emergencies, aminophylline's use as a second-line agent has been well established.

Obtaining a Therapeutic Level

One drawback to theophylline is that a certain amount must be present to achieve an effect. This has been termed a therapeutic level (10–20 mg of the drug per liter of blood). Some patients, however, may benefit from lower levels. To achieve the therapeutic level, a certain dosage must be administered. Dosing is based on the patient's body weight and when given by mouth may require several adjustments based on blood test results before the achievement of a patient's daily maintenance dose. When theophylline is given by mouth, an effect may be achieved in approximately one hour, but it may require two to three days to achieve the desired maintenance level. With intravenous administration of aminophylline, a "loading dose" is usually given over thirty minutes, followed by a constant infusion. Blood levels are again required to adjust the intravenous drip. Compared to the rapidly acting β-agonists, theophylline is both weaker and slower in producing bronchodilatation. Note, however, that when theophylline is given at the same time that the patient is receiving the β-agonist, the effect of the two drugs together may be greater than when given alone.

Adverse Effects of Theophylline

Besides the considerations already described, theophylline may have significant side effects, often related to high blood levels, but some patients may experience adverse effects from small dosages, including stomach and bowel upset, rapid or irregular heartbeat, insomnia, nervousness, urinary frequency, and headache. Some of these effects may be prevented or reduced by avoiding caffeine, which is structurally similar to theophylline; this explains why coffee often has been noted to relieve asthma. Patients should be advised to avoid or reduce caffeine in their diets while receiving theophylline.

Children and Theophylline. One disturbing but controversial side effect has been noted in children—a possible adverse effect on learning and behavior has been raised by some studies. There are conflicting results with other studies that have not demonstrated these effects. At this time, theophylline should be used with caution in young children. Careful monitoring for changes in behavior patterns and learning must be performed.

Overdosage. In excessive or toxic dosages, theophylline may cause nausea, vomiting, irregular heart rhythms, and seizures. Theophylline should never be used without direction and supervision from the physician. Fatalities have been reported in asthmatics that have overused over-the-counter asthma medications that contain theophylline. These over-the-counter preparations have been withdrawn by the FDA.

Drugs That Interact with Theophylline

Another important consideration when patients receive theophylline is the potential for drug interaction, which may result in higher blood levels or toxicity from theophylline. One major group of drugs that can interact with theophylline are certain antibiotics, including erythromycin, clarithromycin (Biaxin), ciprofloxacin (Cipro), levafloxacin (Levaquin), olfloxacin (Floxin), and telithromycin (Ketek). In addition, the widely prescribed stomach medication cimetadine (Tagamet) may also interact with theophylline. One of the anti-leukotrienes, zileuton (Zyflo), has also been found to interact with theophylline. Fortunately, many other antibiotics, stomach medications, and anti-leukotrienes are compatible with theophylline. In instances where one of the drugs that may interact with theophylline must be given, a reduction in the theophylline dosage may be made in order to avoid toxicity. A simple rule is to cut in half the total daily dose whenever receiving one of the above medications mentioned here. It also is vital to monitor blood levels in that situation.

Factors That Affect Theophylline Breakdown

Other factors may contribute to slower breakdown or clearance of theophylline, such as age, liver disease, and heart disease. Elderly patients have been found to clear theophylline more slowly. Patients with diseases of the liver as well as those with congestive heart failure also have been found to have slower metabolism of theophylline. In these groups, lower dosages of theophylline should be given.

Some drugs may accelerate clearance of theophylline from the body. Cigarette and marijuana smokers are often found to clear theophylline more rapidly than nonsmokers and may need their dosages increased. Two medications used for epilepsy, phenytoin (Dilantin) and phenobarbital, may also increase breakdown of theophylline.

Bronchodilator Drugs: Anticholinergic Drugs

For thousands of years it has been observed that anticholinergic drugs have beneficial effects on many patients with respiratory diseases. In fact, many ancient herbal preparations have been found to include atropine (from leaves of the *Atropa belladonna* plant) and stramonium (from the plant *Datura stramonium*). Stramonium cigarettes were commonly smoked in the late nineteenth century for relief of asthma.

How Anticholinergic Agents Work

The action of the anticholinergic agent is believed to be primarily on the tone of the bronchial wall muscle. This muscle tone is thought to be controlled in part by the vagus nerve, a component of the nervous pathway called the cholinergic nervous system. Cholinergic receptors coexist in bronchial wall muscle with the adrenergic receptors. When the cholinergic receptor is stimulated, the activity of the vagus nerve is reduced, resulting in relaxation of the bronchial muscle and bronchodilatation.

Atropine

Physicians have long used atropine for patients with breathing disorders, including asthma. Until recently, however, use of atropine and similar agents has been limited by the total body absorption of these medications, their short duration of action, and their side effects. One disturbing adverse effect is drying of secretions in the respiratory tract. In bronchial asthma this drying may result in increased "plugging" of the bronchial tubes, thereby worsening the attack. Other adverse effects include difficulty with urination (retention), visual changes including blurring of vision and worsening of narrow-angle glaucoma, mental changes including agitation, and dry mouth. It is also important to note that the benefit of these drugs in bronchial asthma was mild and that they were regarded as weak bronchodilators.

Ipratropium Bromide

The introduction of an anticholinergic drug, ipratropium bromide (Atrovent HFA), that was not absorbed to any degree into the total body circulation has permitted the use of this agent in diseases characterized by bronchoconstriction. Due to the extremely small amount of absorption of this drug, no drying effect on bronchial mucus has been noted. Ipratropium bromide (Atrovent HFA) is available as an aerosol medication for MDIs and in solution for nebulization. The recommended MDI dosage is two puffs every six hours. It should be noted that ipratropium bromide has a slow onset of action that may not peak for sixty minutes. The nebulizer solution may be combined with solutions of the β-adrenergic agonists such as albuterol (Duoneb), and a combination MDI (Combivent) is also available.

Ipratropium bromide has not been approved by the FDA for relief of an acute asthmatic attack, but one study of this medication combined with albuterol in an emergency setting found fewer hospitalizations and greater improvement in pulmonary function when compared to albuterol alone.

Tiotropium Bromide

Tiotropium bromide (Spiriva) is a long-acting anticholinergic agent that is many times more potent than ipratropium bromide. It is administered once a day as a powder in a single-dose DPI. The role of tiotropium bromide in asthma management is unknown at this time.

Better Drugs for Emphysema and Chronic Bronchitis

In bronchial asthma the role of the cholinergic system is minor, and, therefore, the effect of anticholinergic drugs is weak compared to β-adrenergic agonists. The anticholinergic agents have no anti-inflammatory effects and no effect on the late phase of bronchial asthma or on bronchial hyperresponsiveness. However, anticholinergic agents are of much greater value for patients with emphysema and chronic bronchitis where it is clear that the vagal cholinergic tone plays a greater role in bronchoconstriction. Those patients with bronchial asthma who have components of emphysema and chronic bronchitis from cigarette abuse or recurrent infection may be good subjects for a trial of ipratropium bromide or tiotropium bromide, but this trial should only occur after primary use of β_2-adrenergic agonists.

Adverse Effects

Adverse effects of ipratropium bromide and tiotropium bromide are few. Small numbers of patients have noted dry mouth, a bitter taste, and headache. Rare reports of increased wheezing after use of the nebulizer solution have been noted. Patients with narrow-angle glaucoma and enlargement of the prostate gland should avoid these agents.

Anti-Inflammatory Drugs: Inhaled Corticosteroids

With greater emphasis being placed on the inflammatory nature of bronchial asthma, the anti-inflammatory agents have achieved greater importance in treatment. The most effective of these agents are corticosteroids, limited to oral or injectable forms until an inhalation form became available. The topically active inhaled steroids have radically changed and improved the treatment of bronchial asthma. Patients who would have previously been dependent on oral steroids with serious lifetime consequences have been able to be maintained on the spray with few side effects. Those patients with milder forms of asthma but who overuse bronchodilator drugs have been able to decrease their consumption of these agents, reducing the adverse effects of these drugs and perhaps avoiding fatal attacks.

Inhaled corticosteroids have reduced the frequency of asthma attacks as well as emergency room visits and hospitalizations for the treatment of severe asthma.

How They Work

Corticosteroids reduce inflammation in the bronchial tubes. Steroids prevent the late phase response and reduce bronchial hyperresponsiveness. The inhaled corticosteroids beclomethasone dipropionate (QVAR), triamcinolone acetonide (Azmacort), flunisolide (Aerobid), budesonide (Pulmicort), fluticasone (Flovent), and mometasone (Asmanex) are "topically active" and achieve their effect on the surface of the bronchial lining. Many of these same agents are used as creams or ointments for skin conditions. If you visualize the lining of the bronchial tube in asthma to be red and inflamed, then the application of the steroid spray is not unlike applying a steroid cream to a skin rash. The results may be a dramatic reduction in inflammation and irritability.

It must be emphasized that for corticosteroids to be effective they must be administered regularly. Too often patients may abandon a steroid inhaler before it has a chance to work. Compared to the β-adrenergic agonists, corticosteroids do not have an immediate effect and cannot rapidly reduce symptoms. For this reason patients may stop this important medication before it has had an adequate trial. Remember that the primary purpose of corticosteroid sprays is prevention. If used correctly these agents may provide long-term control over asthma. In addition, early use of inhaled corticosteroids may prevent permanent changes ("remodeling") that may occur in the bronchial tubes of patients with asthma. Another major benefit of the regular use of inhaled corticosteroid sprays is the reduced need for β_2-agonists, which is extremely important in view of the detrimental effects noted from their overuse.

Specific Agents

Table 4.3 lists the inhaled corticosteroids, their brand names, and the forms that are available. Beclomethasone dipropionate, triamcinolone acetonide, budesonide, fluticasone propionate, mometasone, and flunisolide are available in the United States. Budesonide (Pulmicort Turbuhaler), fluticasone propionate (Flovent Rotadisk), and mometasone (Asmanex) are available in multidose DPI dispensers. Fluticasone propionate is also available as an MDI

Table 4.3   Inhaled Corticosteroids

Drug	Brand Name	Strength μg/puff	Form	Comment
Beclomethasone	QVAR	40, 80	MDI	HFA, small particle size
Budesonide	Pulmicort	200	DPI	Turbuhaler
	Pulmicort Respules		Nebulizer	0.25 mg, 0.5 mg
Flunisolide	Aerobid	250	MDI	
	Aerobid-M	250	MDI	Mint flavor
Fluticasone	Flovent HFA	44, 110, 220	MDI	HFA
	Flovent Rotadisk	50, 100, 250	DPI	
Mometasone	Asmanex	220	DPI	Twisthaler, once-a-day
Triamcinolone	Azmacort	100	MDI	Built-in spacer

(Flovent HFA) and in combination with a long-acting β_2-agonist, salmeterol, in a multidose DPI form (Advair Diskus). Budesonide (Pulmicort Respules) is the only inhaled corticosteroid available for use in a nebulizer.

Dosage and Administration

Inhaled corticosteroids may be given in varying dosages depending on individual patients. A common starting dose would be between 100 and 400 micrograms (μg) per day. High doses (600–2,000 μg) may be necessary for control of severe asthma. Inhaled corticosteroids are usually given twice a day. Mometasone (Asmanex) has been shown to be effective when given once a day in the evening to stable patients.

Current information suggests that the inhaled corticosteroids are not equivalent on a per puff or microgram (μg) basis. Fluticasone propionate and mometasone appear to be the most potent agents in laboratory studies. Although these laboratory studies appear to correlate with increased effectiveness in patients, direct comparison of all six agents is lacking. The delivery systems used to administer inhaled corticosteroid may affect the effectiveness of the specific medication. For example, when budesonide is administered as a DPI (Pulmicort Turbuhaler), twice the amount of medication is delivered when compared to the MDI. Budesonide is only available in the DPI form in the United States.

Beclomethasone HFA (QVAR) has been compared to beclomethasone CFC. The small particle size of the HFA preparation produces greater delivery of this medication to the lungs with less deposition in the mouth and throat. Mometasone DPI (Asmanex) has been found to be more effective than budesonide DPI (Pulmicort) and as effective as fluticasone (Flovent). Fluticasone is available in three dosages (44, 110, and 220 µg per puff), which allows increased flexibility in adjusting the appropriate dosage for the individual patient. Table 4.4 shows daily dosages for inhaled corticosteroids.

"High-Dose" Inhalers. In view of the large number of sprays needed on a daily basis for many patients, "high-dose" sprays are available with up to 250 µg per puff of corticosteroid. Usually these inhalers allow patients with stable asthma to be maintained on two puffs twice a day. Mometasone (Asmanex) dispenses 220 µg per activation of a multidose DPI. Stable patients may be maintained on as little as one dose per day of this medication.

Adverse Effects and How to Prevent Them

The primary side effect of inhaled corticosteroids is development of a yeast infection known as candidiasis in the mouth or throat. With large numbers of puffs from the "low-dose" inhaler or the use of the "high-dose" preparation, there is a greater risk of this infection. This is a local infection, and the rare instances of its spreading outside the mouth have typically occurred in patients with lowered immunity who took no precautionary steps. Several preventive steps can be taken to avoid the infection, including rinsing the mouth and spitting after spraying. If unable to rinse, the

Table 4.4   Comparative Daily Dosages for Inhaled Corticosteroids

Drug	Low Dose	Medium Dose	High Dose
Beclomethasone HFA (QVAR) 40 or 80 μg/puff	**Adult:** 80–240 μg ***Child:** 80–160 μg	**Adult:** 240–480 μg **Child:** 160–320 μg	**Adult:** >480 μg **Child:** >320 μg
Budesonide DPI (Pulmicort) 200 μg/inhalation	**Adult:** 200–600 μg **Child:** 200–400 μg	**Adult:** 600–1,200 μg **Child:** 400–800 μg	**Adult:** >1,200 μg **Child:** >800 μg
Budesonide Suspension (Pulmicort Respules) for nebulizer	**Child:** 0.5 mg	**Child:** 1.0 mg	**Child:** 2.0 mg
Flunisolide (Aerobid) 250 μg/puff	**Adult:** 500–1,000 μg **Child:** 500–750 μg	**Adult:** 1,000–2,000 μg **Child:** 1,000–1,250 μg	**Adult:** >2,000 μg **Child:** >1,250 μg
Fluticasone HFA (Flovent-HFA) 44, 110, 220 μg/puff	**Adult:** 88–264 μg **Child:** 88–176 μg	**Adult:** 264–660 μg **Child:** 176–440 μg	**Adult:** >660 μg **Child:** >440 μg
Fluticasone DPI (Flovent Rotadisk) 50, 100, 250 μg/inhalation	**Adult:** 100–300 μg **Child:** 100–200 μg	**Adult:** 300–600 μg **Child:** 200–400 μg	**Adult:** >600 μg **Child:** >400 μg
Mometasone (Asmanex) 220 μg/inhalation	**Adult:** 220–440 μg	**Adult:** 440–880 μg	**Adult:** >880 μg
Triamcinolone (Azmacort) 100 μg/puff	**Adult:** 400–1,000 μg **Child:** 400–800 μg	**Adult:** 1,000–2,000 μg **Child:** 800–1,200 μg	**Adult:** >2,000 μg **Child:** >1,200 μg

*Children twelve years of age or under

patient may simply drink, flushing residual medication away from the mouth and throat. Passage through the digestive tract leads to rapid breakdown of the drug but rinsing is still preferred. Another extremely helpful step in administering inhaled steroid aimed at reducing the risk of yeast infection is a spacer. This simple device improves delivery of the steroid to the lung as well as reducing the amount likely to be deposited in the mouth and throat. Triamcinolone acetonide (Azmacort) incorporates a spacer in its MDI.

If candidiasis is discovered, treatment should be administered promptly, consisting usually of an antifungal agent (nystatin, clotrimazole) prepared as an oral suspension or as a lozenge. It is rare that development of an oral yeast infection will recur, prompting discontinuation of inhaled steroids. In patients with recurrent yeast infection a switch to another anti-inflammatory agent such as an anti-leukotriene (Singulair, Accolate), cromolyn sodium (Intal), or nedocromil (Tilade) is indicated.

Another infrequent side effect of inhaled steroids is an effect on the voice, usually noted as hoarseness that may be alleviated with a spacer and by a temporary reduction in dosage. Patients who complain of changes in voice should have a careful examination of the vocal cords to ensure that there is no other explanation for the abnormality.

Are Inhaled Steroid Sprays Really Safe?

There is often great fear on the part of patients when the discussion of asthma medication turns to corticosteroids. This may explain why these agents are often underused. It is common to associate inhaled steroids with the side effects of oral or injected steroid drugs. Inhaled steroids are not absorbed in appreciable amounts into the bloodstream and total body, and they are not the body-building steroids that have received so much media attention. The minor and infrequent side effects already noted are usually not significant and rarely cause a patient to stop treatment. In children the normal dosages prescribed have not been found to produce significant side effects. Higher dosages in children may have effects on bone growth, but these usually can be avoided with the addition of a long-acting β_2-agonist and either an anti-leukotriene, cromolyn, nedocromil, or low-dose theophylline.

The effectiveness of inhaled corticosteroids in the control of asthma has been demonstrated in a large number of studies. These agents have been shown to reduce the frequency of asthmatic attacks, decrease β_2-agonist use, improve lung function, and reduce the number of hospitalizations for severe asthma. Corticosteroids are the most potent anti-inflammatory agent available for the treatment of asthma.

A study of adults receiving high doses of inhaled corticosteroids (1,500–1,600 μg per day) revealed a greater risk for the development of glaucoma in asthmatics, sixty-six years of age and older. This study also demonstrated that there was no increased risk of glaucoma from the use of nasal steroid sprays or from inhaled corticosteroids at lower dosages. Patients receiving high-dose inhaled steroids for less than three months did not have an increased glaucoma risk.

An increased risk of the development of cataracts in older asthmatics that used inhaled corticosteroids has also been reported. This study also suggested greater risk with high doses and prolonged use of inhaled corticosteroids. Studies of children and young adults receiving inhaled corticosteroids have not revealed early cataract formation. The risk of cataract formation can be reduced by not smoking, limiting ultraviolet light exposure with sunglasses, taking a multivitamin tablet daily, and eating at least three servings per day of fresh fruits or green leafy vegetables. Adult asthmatics who are receiving inhaled corticosteroids, especially those age sixty-five and older, should have periodic eye examinations.

Reduce Inhaled Corticosteroid Dosages

In order to reduce the risk of adverse effects of inhaled corticosteroids, the daily dosage should be reduced when good control of the asthma is achieved. In general, it is best to use higher dosages initially to achieve control and then to "step down" to moderate or low doses. Several recent studies have demonstrated that the combination of a long-acting bronchodilator (salmeterol or formoterol) or the addition of an anti-leukotriene or oral theophylline to an inhaled corticosteroid results in fewer symptoms in patients with moderate asthma. By adding these agents, higher dosages of inhaled corticosteroids in these patients may be avoided.

How Soon Should I See an Effect?

A reasonable trial of an inhaled corticosteroid will often require two to three weeks. At that point dosage may have to be adjusted to achieve a significant effect over an additional two to three weeks.

How Long Must I Remain on My Steroid Spray?

Long-term studies have determined that the benefits of inhaled topical corticosteroids are not maximized for periods approaching one year of use. There is clearly a slow onset of action, and patients who abandon their medication at three months or less are deprived of further benefits from continued use. "Can I be cured of my asthma by a steroid spray?" is a frequent question asked by patients. The answer is that a cure is unlikely and infrequent. Individual patients treated for at least one year with a steroid spray have been able to discontinue medication and remain well, but long-term follow-up is lacking in these patients. It should be emphasized that bronchial asthma is usually a chronic disease and treatment is often for life.

Do I Have to Use My B-Agonist Spray Before My Steroid Spray?

It has been a common and widespread practice to give a short-acting β_2-agonist before the inhaled steroid spray to facilitate the entry and penetration of the steroid medication. In stable patients, however, it has been demonstrated that this is not necessary. Such patients may use their steroid spray alone and achieve equal delivery of medication. Patients who are wheezing or who note increased cough after their steroid spray may be helped by premedication with the β-agonist. If the two agents are used together, it is important to allow five to ten minutes between them, enough time for the β-agonist to achieve significant bronchodilation before the steroid is applied.

Anti-Inflammatory Drugs: Systemic Corticosteroids

Before introduction of inhaled corticosteroids in the 1970s, anti-inflammatory drugs were limited to oral or injectable preparations that produced total body or systemic effects. Many patients with bronchial asthma became steroid dependent for life and developed serious side effects. Although inhaled corticosteroids have spared many patients this "life sentence" or allowed many to reduce their steroid dosages, systemic corticosteroids are still often required to treat acute and severe bronchial asthma.

When Should Systemic Steroids Be Used?

In patients with severe attacks who are already receiving bronchodilator and anti-inflammatory therapy, a course of an oral steroid such as prednisone, prednisolone, or methylprednisolone will be necessary. Patients who require emergency room care and/or hospitalization will often require intravenous preparations of hydrocortisone (Solucortef) or methylprednisolone (Solumedrol). In treating severe asthma the most common error is to undertreat with smaller dosages of steroid than necessary. This error often arises from the concern that adverse side effects will develop, although a short course of corticosteroids usually produces few such effects. If adverse effects do develop, they are usually transient and quickly resolve after the course of steroids is concluded.

Dosages of Oral Corticosteroids

A typical short course of oral steroid in the setting of a severe attack resistant to the patient's maintenance and contingent medications would start at a dosage of prednisone (or an equivalent dosage of methylprednisolone) of 40–60 mg a day. Patients with more severe disease and a history of requiring courses of oral steroid are more likely to require the higher dosage. Depending on the severity of the attack, this dosage may be maintained from one to seven days before it is reduced and the total course may extend from approximately one to three weeks. This tapering is especially necessary for the longer courses to allow the adrenal gland to function normally.

Considering the Adrenal Gland

The adrenal gland produces the body's own supply of cortisone. When this gland recognizes that corticosteroid is present in the bloodstream in quantities greater than usual, it stops its own production. This is called adrenal suppression, and the state of inactivity is termed "adrenal insufficiency." In this state, the absence of cortisone under stressful conditions may produce low blood pressure and shock. The tapering of steroid dosages allows the gland to recover function. For extremely brief courses, however, tapering is not necessary.

In-Hospital Use of Steroids

Patients who are hospitalized with severe attacks are usually treated with intravenous methylprednisolone (Solumedrol) in dosages varying between 40 mg and 60 mg intravenously every six hours. This dosage is usually maintained for one to three days, and then tapered with transfer to an oral corticosteroid. The taper of the oral steroid may extend another one to three weeks. With high doses of intravenous or oral corticosteroid being administered, the addition of the inhaled steroid does not contribute significantly to treatment. Inhaled corticosteroids are not as valuable in treating acute attacks and should be considered primarily preventive medications. Therefore, they are usually introduced or restarted after the acute attack symptoms have greatly improved. Due to slow onset of action it is helpful to overlap the lower tapering dosages of the oral steroid and the inhaled form. A good starting point is when the oral taper reaches 15 mg of prednisone or its equivalent.

Changing from Oral to Inhaled Steroids

The transition from oral to inhaled corticosteroid must be closely supervised. Patients who have been maintained on oral corticosteroids for long periods or who have received frequent courses may have adrenal insufficiency. This would be less likely in patients who had been maintained on alternate-day steroids. Laboratory testing can be performed by the physician to determine the state of the adrenal gland. As the oral dosage of corticosteroid is reduced and eliminated and the inhaled steroids are utilized, it is best to assume that adrenal insufficiency exists for a period of six to twelve months after the last oral dosage has been given. If a medical illness develops, such as influenza, it is advisable to administer a dosage of oral corticosteroid that would equal what the adrenal gland would normally produce.

Intramuscular Injection of Steroids

Another method of administration of corticosteroid is by intramuscular injection. Triamcinolone acetonide (Kenalog) is one steroid that can be given on a monthly basis by this route. A recent study demonstrated that this medication could provide maintenance control equal to that achieved by oral corticosteroid. Intramuscular injection may have some value in patients who find it difficult to follow a tapering oral schedule but certainly carries a high risk of total body side effects. One additional adverse effect that has been noted with intramuscular corticosteroid is atrophy or wasting of the muscle at the site of injection.

What Time Should I Take My Oral Steroid Dosage?

Because the greatest quantity of the body's corticosteroid is produced in the early morning hours, it has been common practice to prescribe dosing in the morning. Patients with nocturnal asthma have often "split" the total daily dose and taken half in the morning and half at bedtime. Research has demonstrated that better control of asthma results from patients receiving their entire daily dosage at 3 p.m. This may be due partly to the slow onset of action of several hours after a dosage is ingested. This slow onset is also important when initiating treatment for a severe attack. If there is delay in the decision to give steroids, this is further compounded by delayed onset of action. With the help of peak flow measurements the decision to treat should be straightforward.

Alternate-Day Steroids. Another approach to the administration of oral corticosteroids is alternate-day dosing. This approach has been found to reduce adverse effects, particularly adrenal insufficiency. Unfortunately this "day on, day off" approach is not strong enough to control the acute asthmatic attack. It may be helpful, however, in maintenance control of bronchial asthma when an inhaled corticosteroid has not achieved adequate control. Patients with severe disease may still experience difficulty on the "day off" and require small daily dosing for better control.

Adverse Effects of Systemic Steroids

Any adverse effects of corticosteroids are directly related to how long they are administered and in what dosage. The greater the dosage the likelier the development of side effects, especially if sustained at high dosage for a prolonged period (months to years). One of the most serious side effects is development of adrenal insufficiency. In this setting the careful administration of steroid is essential since without the patient's daily dosage there is a risk of low blood pressure and collapse. This is particularly important when the body is placed under stress as in an infection, since the adrenal gland is responsible for maintaining normal body chemistry under severe conditions.

Other adverse effects of systemic corticosteroids include high blood pressure, diabetes, stomach ulcer, osteoporosis, mental changes, fluid retention, thinning of the skin with easy bruising, accelerated cataract formation, obesity, and mental changes. There may also be hormonal changes that affect the menstrual cycle. Over prolonged periods increased fat may be deposited in the liver with enlargement of this organ. All these effects are particularly damaging to the older population of asthmatics who may already have some of these problems. In these patients the underlying illness is often worsened, as in the patient whose diabetes was previously controlled by diet but who on corticosteroids must now take oral medication or insulin. It is clear that in individual patients the adverse effects of oral corticosteroids may be severe and in some cases cause ailments that the patient feels are "worse than my asthma."

How Can I Avoid Side Effects of Corticosteroids? Any time corticosteroids are prescribed orally or by injection, it must be clear that they are absolutely necessary. This is best determined by the physician in communication with the patient with readings of spirometry or peak flow. Patients should have clear guidelines from their physicians concerning their use of steroids and always consult with their doctors before using steroids. In emergencies where communication is delayed, the patient should follow dosage guidelines already agreed on and report to the physician as soon as possible.

When steroids are prescribed they must be given in sufficient dosage to alleviate the attack in conjunction with other medications. One common error is to prolong treatment unnecessarily. Reducing dosage when it is appropriate reduces the magnitude of any side effects. Home monitoring by peak flow can be invaluable in deciding how often and how much of a reduction in corticosteroid is possible. If prolonged steroid use is necessary, the lowest possible but still effective dosage should be given. An alternate-day approach may also be tried.

Preparing for Side Effects. When corticosteroids are prescribed it is best to prepare for side effects, including careful monitoring of calorie intake as well as the amount of salt and fluids consumed in an attempt to reduce weight gain and swelling (edema). Increased exercise, hopefully permitted by reduced asthmatic symptoms, can be extremely helpful in slowing weight gain. Exercise is important since steroids may cause myopathy, or muscle weakness. Since steroids cause an increased loss of potassium from the body, a diet rich in potassium is helpful. Citrus fruits and their juices as well as bananas also increase potassium intake. Increased calcium intake with vitamin D may help reduce bone loss. In women with osteoporosis, the use of a bisphosphonate medication in conjunction with calcium and vitamin D is more effective in preventing bone loss than supplements of calcium and vitamin D alone. Patients with mild diabetes or a tendency to high blood sugar should increase restriction of their diets when they are placed on steroids. These patients must have their blood sugars closely monitored and may require treatment such as oral hypoglycemic agents or insulin.

Preventing Osteoporosis. Corticosteroids impair bone health when taken orally or by injection on a regular basis. They interfere with calcium absorption from foods and increase the amount of calcium lost through the kidneys. When calcium levels fall, calcium must be mobilized from the bone to return blood levels to normal, thereby reducing bone mass (causing osteoporosis). Corticosteroids also activate cells that break down bone called osteoclasts and inhibit bone-forming cells (osteoblasts). The end result is bone breakdown and increased risk of fractures. Another important steroid effect on bone is through the reduction in production of sex hormones. Steroids suppress both estrogen and testosterone, resulting in reduced bone density in men and women. Steroid-induced osteoporosis is not associated with aging and may even affect children.

Patients receiving oral corticosteroids should consume at least 1,500 milligrams of calcium and 800 international units of vitamin D a day, either through diet or supplements. In addition, patients should exercise regularly and avoid smoking and excessive alcohol use. Men receiving corticosteroids should have their testosterone measured and may benefit from replacement therapy. A bone density measurement is recommended for anyone starting a long course of corticosteroid. Estrogen may be recommended for women at menopause, but prolonged use is not currently recommended. Several medications known as bisphosphonates (Fosamax, Actonel, Boniva, Didrocal) are available. They increase bone mass by blocking osteoclasts, which resorb bone. These medications may have significant adverse effects on the digestive tract so they may not be tolerated by everyone. In this situation, a hormone known as calcitonin-salmon (Miacalcin), which increases bone mass and is delivered as a nasal spray, may be substituted. Another option is an injectable medication, teriparatide (Forteo), which is a man-made form of a hormone produced by the parathyroid gland. This medication forms new bone, increases bone density and strength, and reduces the risk of fractures. Forteo is available in a self-injector form and is reserved for patients with osteoporosis who are considered at high risk for fractures.

Protecting the Stomach. To minimize stomach irritation, steroids should always be taken with food. Antacids may also be given if acidity increases but are best not taken simultaneously with the steroid since its absorption is decreased. Patients with histories of stomach ulcer are best placed on a regimen of anti-ulcer medication while they are receiving corticosteroids. This may include one of two groups of medications (H2 antagonists that reduce the amount of stomach acid and/or proton-pump inhibitors that completely shut down acid production).

When Side Effects Cannot Be Prevented. Unfortunately, some side effects cannot be avoided or minimized. Patients on prolonged corticosteroids should have frequent eye exams to check for accelerated formation of cataracts or increased glaucoma. In addition, there is little that can be done for the increased fragility of the skin or increased bruising other than finding the lowest maintenance dose possible or hopefully discontinuing the oral steroid successfully. The mental changes also cannot be avoided other than by lowering dosages. The initial high dosages may result in euphoria and, rarely, psychosis. Steroid withdrawal may produce depression. It is helpful to be aware of these possible effects, allowing the patient and family to adjust accordingly.

Anti-Inflammatory Drugs: Anti-Leukotrienes

The redefinition of asthma as an inflammatory disease of the bronchial tubes has resulted in research focused on drug therapies that target inflammation. One result of this research was the introduction of the anti-leukotriene agents. These oral medications represent another option in the effort to better control bronchial asthma.

What Is a Leukotriene?

A variety of cells are involved in the development of inflammation of the airways in asthma. These cells release chemical substances called mediators that promote inflammation. Leukotrienes are one group of these irritating chemicals. They are produced when the walls of mast cells break down during allergic and asthmatic attacks. After the leukotrienes are released, they must bind to receptors in the bronchial tubes to produce their effects. Levels of leukotrienes may remain elevated for weeks after an asthmatic attack. Medications that block the actions of leukotrienes have been shown to reduce the number of asthmatic attacks and to improve breathing function.

Patients with mild to moderate asthma who have been treated with an anti-leukotriene agent have been shown to reduce their use of β_2-agonists and to require less frequent courses of oral corticosteroids. The anti-leukotrienes offer an alternative to the inhaled corticosteroids or may be used to reduce high dosages of these agents. It should be noted, however, that as a group, inhaled corticosteroids have greater anti-inflammatory effects than anti-leukotrienes. In patients with severe asthma, anti-leukotrienes may allow reduction or withdrawal of oral corticosteroids. These agents also appear to be particularly effective in asthmatics with exercise-induced asthma (see Chapter 9) and aspirin hypersensitivity (see Chapter 11) and are the anti-inflammatory agent of choice in these patients. The oral dosing of these medications may make them more convenient for patients, improving compliance with treatment. Anti-leukotrienes are also approved for the treatment of allergic rhinitis (hay fever). Three anti-leukotriene medications are currently available: montelukast (Singulair), zafirlukast (Accolate), and zileuton (Zyflo).

Montelukast

Montelukast (Singulair) is a leukotriene antagonist that acts by binding to the leukotriene receptor in the bronchial tubes and nasal passages. The dosage for those age fifteen years and older is one 10 mg tablet daily, taken at bedtime. It may be taken with or without food. Montelukast also has been approved for use in children. The dosage for children six to fourteen years of age is one 5 mg chewable tablet daily. For children one to five years of age, the dosage is 4 mg given as granules that may be mixed with applesauce, carrots, rice, or ice cream.

Adverse Effects. Montelukast is extremely well tolerated in both adults and children with infrequent significant side effects and without drug interactions. A small percentage of patients may notice a queasy stomach and about 11 percent of patients complain of headache.

Since the introduction of montelukast, a small number of patients have been reported who developed a rare illness known as the Churg-Strauss Syndrome (CSS). This illness is characterized by severe asthma (requiring oral corticosteroids), elevation of allergy cells known as eosinophils, and inflammation of small blood vessels (vasculitis), with effects throughout many parts of the body including the skin, lung, and kidneys. In some of the patients who developed CSS on Singulair, steroid dosages were reduced after the introduction of this drug, raising the possibility that this medication simply "unmasked" the illness by allowing physicians to reduce steroids.

Zileuton

Zileuton (Zyflo) reduces leukotriene production by inhibiting an enzyme (5-lipoxygenase) involved in its production. The dosage of zileuton is 600 mg taken by mouth four times a day, with or without food. After three months, the dosage may be reduced to 600 mg twice a day. A response to this medication is usually noted after two weeks, with maximal effect achieved in one to four months.

A twice-a-day preparation of zileuton is currently in development.

Adverse Effects. Approximately 4 percent of patients taking zileuton will develop abnormal liver function tests. These blood tests should be evaluated prior to starting zileuton and periodically during treatment. Seven liver function tests are recommended in the first year. A drug interaction between zileuton and theophylline has been well documented. A good general rule is to reduce the daily theophylline dosage by one-third when starting zileuton and to monitor theophylline levels.

Zafirlukast

Zafirlukast (Accolate) was the first anti-leukotriene agent to be marketed in the United States. This agent is a leukotriene antagonist that acts by binding to the leukotriene receptor. The dosage of zafirlukast is 20 mg twice a day, taken on an empty stomach (an hour before or two hours after a meal). Zafirlukast may produce beneficial effects in days but requires at least a two-week period to determine a response to treatment.

Adverse Effects. Zafirlukast is usually well tolerated. Headache and nausea have been noted infrequently and rarely require discontinuation of the drug. Six out of the first 270,000 Americans who took zafirlukast were reported to have developed the Churg-Strauss Syndrome. This is similar to the finding of CSS in patients receiving montelukast and may have occurred as a result of a reduction in steroid dosage. A direct, allergic reaction in some patients is also possible. Physicians are advised to reduce oral corticosteroids carefully in previously steroid-dependent asthmatics.

A drug interaction with warfarin (Coumadin), a commonly prescribed blood thinner, has been observed with zafirlukast. Patients receiving this blood thinner who require an anti-leukotriene agent should receive either zileuton or montelukast.

Anti-Inflammatory Drugs: Cromolyn Sodium

Cromolyn sodium, a derivative of khellin, an Egyptian herbal remedy, is an anti-inflammatory agent that may be used as an alternative to inhaled corticosteroids. In severe patients, cromolyn sodium (Intal) may be used in conjunction with steroids. Since its introduction, cromolyn has been a helpful drug for childhood asthmatics. From this early application it has been incorrectly assumed that it was a poor drug for adults, particularly those without allergic characteristics. Many studies, however, have documented that cromolyn may be an effective drug for asthmatics of all ages, even in patients with "intrinsic" asthma. It is also clear that cromolyn does not work for all patients. Like the inhaled corticosteroids, it is slow acting and, therefore, requires a trial of three to six weeks to assess response. Because of this, many patients abandon this drug before it has had an adequate trial. Another drawback is that cromolyn must be administered several times a day, which reduces patient compliance.

How Does Cromolyn Work?

It is not clear how cromolyn sodium reduces inflammation. Some evidence has pointed to an action on inflammatory and allergy cells that prevents release of irritating chemicals that cause inflammation. There may also be an antagonistic action on nervous stimulation that prevents bronchoconstriction and reflex cough. Cromolyn has been demonstrated to prevent both the immediate and late reactions of asthma as well as exercise-induced asthma in many patients.

How Cromolyn Is Supplied and Used

Cromolyn sodium was initially made available as a powder for inhalation. Unfortunately, this produced considerable coughing and wheezing. It is currently also available as an aerosol for MDIs and in solution for nebulization. When used for nebulization it may be combined with a β_2-adrenergic agonist. The recommended dosage is two puffs four times a day from an MDI or 20 mg in solution via a nebulizer, also four times a day.

Cromolyn is not an effective drug for acute asthmatic attacks and, similar to inhaled corticosteroids, must be used as a preventive maintenance drug. For this reason it is best not to start cromolyn during an acute attack. It can be introduced toward the end of an oral steroid taper similar to the way that the inhaled corticosteroids are started. Also, like the inhaled corticosteroids, cromolyn can be used alone and does not necessarily require premedication with a β-agonist.

Adverse Effects of Cromolyn

Besides being an effective drug, cromolyn has an extremely low incidence of side effects, which explains its frequent use in children. As research has shown that inhaled corticosteroids are generally safe and more effective, cromolyn has become a second-line agent. In those patients with adverse steroid effects cromolyn is an alternative anti-inflammatory agent. There are few adverse effects to speak of. Occasionally, cough and wheezing may result from its inhalation. This can often be prevented with the use of a β-agonist sprayed five to ten minutes before use or given in solution with cromolyn via nebulization. Rarely have total body effects been noted. An extremely small number of patients have noted joint pains and rash, which resolved completely on discontinuation.

Anti-Inflammatory Drugs: Nedocromil Sodium

Nedocromil sodium (Tilade) resembles cromolyn sodium in its effects as an anti-inflammatory. Nedocromil, however, is structurally different from cromolyn sodium and may also prevent the release of irritating chemicals that perpetuate the asthmatic reaction, but its mechanism of action is unknown. It also has effects on the immediate allergic response and the late phase reaction. There is some evidence that nedocromil may be helpful in reducing the number of puffs of inhaled steroids needed to maintain good control of asthma.

How Nedocromil Is Supplied and Used

Nedocromil has been made available in the United States as an aerosol delivered by MDI. Compared with cromolyn sodium, nedocromil appears to be more potent and in a large series of patients has been shown to be slightly more effective. The daily dosage is two puffs four times a day but may be reduced to twice a day in stable patients. Nedrocromil should be regarded as an alternative to inhaled corticosteroids, and cromolyn as a preventive anti-inflammatory. It has no place in the treatment of the acute asthmatic attack and is best introduced toward the end of an oral steroid taper for patients who have suffered an acute episode. Nedocromil also has a slow onset of action and should be given for three to six weeks before judgment is made as to its effectiveness.

Adverse Effects of Nedocromil

Like cromolyn sodium, nedocromil has few total body side effects. Patient acceptance, however, has been affected by a greater incidence of nausea after its use as well as aftertaste and occasionally throat irritation. Rarely, a flushing sensation may be noted after its use. For these reasons, it is unlikely that nedocromil will replace cromolyn. A menthol-flavored version is available in Europe and hopefully will be made available in the United States. It is too early to know if this will overcome some of the adverse effects noted.

Omalizumab

Omalizumab (Xolair) is a recent exciting and unique advance in the treatment of allergic or extrinsic asthma. It is an Immunoglobulin E (IgE) blocker that has a totally different mechanism of action than any other current asthma therapy.

How Does Omalizumab Work?

As noted in Chapter 1, allergic reactions begin with exposure to allergens, which may be inhaled. In a susceptible allergic person this exposure triggers a response of the immune system that leads to the production of a specific IgE. This protein circulates in the blood and attaches itself to the surface of mast cells, which contain irritating chemicals. When the IgE attached to the mast cells combines with the allergen, these cells disintegrate, releasing the chemicals that produce inflammation of the lining of the bronchial tubes and an asthmatic attack is initiated. Omalizumab works by locking on the IgE, preventing its interaction with allergens and the breakdown of mast cells.

In large studies, patients receiving Xolair experienced fewer asthma attacks and reduced their need for other asthma medications including oral and inhaled corticosteroids.

Who Should Receive Omalizumab?

Omalizumab is approved for use in people twelve years of age or older with documented allergies and uncontrolled moderate to severe persistent asthma. These individuals typically are receiving several asthma medications including inhaled and oral corticosteroids but continue to require their emergency or "rescue" short-acting bronchodilator daily. Tests of pulmonary function such as peak flows and spirometry are well below expected values.

Omalizumab may receive FDA approval for use in children by 2008.

How Is Allergy Determined?

In order to qualify for omalizumab, an elevation in blood IgE level must be demonstrated. This is done through a blood test. In addition, the patient must have had positive allergy testing. The tests may also be done through blood sampling (RAST tests) or by allergy skin testing.

How Do I Obtain Omalizumab?

Omalizumab has been restricted to several specialty pharmacies. For you to receive this medication, your doctor must provide one of these pharmacies with a prescription that includes the diagnosis of allergic asthma, what medications you are currently taking, your IgE level, and the positive results of allergy testing. Omalizumab is expensive (approximately $500–$1,000 per month) so the pharmacy will then contact your insurance company to determine coverage. If coverage is approved, the pharmacy will ship the drug to your physician or if you prefer, directly to you.

How Is Omalizumab Given?

This medication is administered by injection under the skin every two to four weeks. The dosage of omalizumab is calculated by an individual's weight and IgE level. The more allergic the person, the higher the amount needed to neutralize the allergy protein. The medication is shipped as a powder, which must be reconstituted with sterile water. Once reconstituted, omalizumab is a viscous liquid. Patients may be taught to self-administer omalizumab, not unlike a diabetic who injects insulin. The first injections are always administered in the doctor's office to look for any adverse effects. In my experience to date, most patients have elected to have their injections in the physician's office. A pre-filled, self-injecting form of omalizumab may be available in 2007, which will likely increase home administration of this medication.

What Are the Side Effects of Omalizumab?

Omalizumab has been well tolerated in the vast majority of the more than thirty thousand patients receiving it in the United States. A severe allergic reaction known as anaphylaxis has been seen in less that 0.1 percent of patients. The most common side effect is injection-site reaction, which may be soreness or itching. One of my patients developed generalized itching, which was treated with an antihistamine taken before the injection.

In early human studies, 0.5 percent of patients receiving omalizumab developed cancer compared with 0.2 percent of patients receiving a placebo injection. This result appears to have been due to the small number of patients in this early study; as additional patients have been added, no increase in the incidence of cancer has been found.

How Soon Should I See an Effect?

To date I have personally treated nearly forty patients with omalizumab. The first patient I treated was Bill, a middle-aged man who had suffered from severe asthma for many years and had required frequent courses of oral corticosteroids. His list of medications stretched over two pages, and he carried with him a bag of aerosol sprays and a portable nebulizer. Bill also suffered from severe hay fever with constant nasal congestion. The day after his first injection, I received a call from him. "Doc, I can breathe through my nose and my chest feels better." When he returned for his second injection, I noticed that he was not carrying that ever-present bag of medicines. "This drug is like a miracle. I don't need my albuterol anymore, and I'm sleeping through the night. Can I stop them all?" We then sat down in my office and made a plan to gradually wean off as many medications as possible, including reducing the number of puffs of the inhaled steroid. Within a few months, Bill was using only a low dose of his inhaler steroid and rarely needed his "rescue" albuterol spray.

Not all patients have had as dramatic a response to omalizumab. The vast majority of patients improve significantly. In some patients, however, it may not be effective and a few of my patients have elected to stop treatment. Of note, in my experience patients with only mild elevations of IgE may do as well with treatment as those with much higher levels.

When Do I Stop Omalizumab?

This medication is designed for maintenance treatment of bronchial asthma. Once a beneficial effect has been determined, treatment should continue on a regular basis. Studies of long-term administration of omalizumab have noted continued improvement even after one year of treatment.

Future Indications

Omalizumab has also been found to be effective in the treatment of allergic rhinitis and may also receive this indication from the FDA. Individuals with severe food allergies, latex allergy, allergic skin rashes, and persistent hives (urticaria) have also been successfully treated with omalizumab, so this medication may also receive these future indications.

Other Asthma Medications

Etanercept (Enbrel)

Etanercept is a drug commonly used to treat rheumatoid arthritis. In small studies, early research has shown that twice-weekly injections of this drug in patients with severe asthma provided significant improvement. Many of these patients who had required oral corticosteroids reported decreased asthma symptoms and improved control despite steroid reduction. Etanercept works by blocking a chemical released by the immune system called tumor necrosis factor alpha (TNF-α). This chemical is not associated with mild asthma, but researchers have found that as the disease becomes severe there is a change that promotes production of TNF-α. Preformed TNF-α has been found in mast cells and may be rapidly released during IgE-mediated allergic and asthmatic reactions.

A recent study has found high levels of TNF-α in patients with severe asthma, resistant to the effects of high-dose corticosteroids. TNF-α appears to play a significant role in producing bronchial hyperresponsiveness, particularly in patients with severe asthma. Larger studies of etanercept and other TNF-α inhibitors in patients with severe asthma are needed to confirm these results. It should be noted that etanercept's effects on the immune system can make a person more susceptible to infections and that there is a risk of developing lymphoma in patients receiving this drug.

Methotrexate

Several trials of methotrexate in patients with severe, often steroid-dependent asthma have taken place. Methotrexate reduces the immune response of the body by reducing the number of white blood cells in tissues. These cells carry the irritating chemicals that can cause inflammation. The use of this drug in asthma stems from its effectiveness in another inflammatory illness, rheumatoid arthritis. Patients with this severe joint disease have often benefited from low-dose (once a week) administration of methotrexate.

Early studies of methotrexate suggested this drug may have a beneficial effect in bronchial asthma, allowing some patients to reduce their steroid requirement. Further studies have not been as positive, and long-term studies of adverse effects in asthmatic patients have not been completed. Since methotrexate may cause pneumonia and scarring of the lungs known as pulmonary fibrosis, its use in patients with underlying lung disease such as asthma may prove hazardous. An additional worrisome side effect is the potential for liver damage. Patients receiving methotrexate must have frequent blood tests for liver function, chest x-rays, and comprehensive pulmonary function tests looking for evidence of fibrosis. Unless further studies show a greater benefit to this drug's use in bronchial asthma, it is likely to be used sparingly.

Cyclosporin A

Other agents that suppress the immune response have also been tried in severe asthma. One of these is cyclosporin A, which has been used to a great extent in preventing rejection of transplanted organs. This agent is active against lymphocytes, white blood cells that are active in asthma. Like methotrexate, studies to date do not show a great enough beneficial effect of cyclosporin A on asthma that would outweigh the risk of side effects on the immune system.

Gold Salts

Gold salts have been administered to asthmatic patients because this drug has benefited patients with rheumatoid arthritis. Small numbers of patients have been treated with gold injections or an oral gold compound called auranofin (Ridaura), and individual patients have been reported to reduce their symptoms and steroid requirements. Studies of large numbers of patients are lacking, and this approach is not without adverse side effects, since gold may also cause pulmonary fibrosis. For these reasons, the use of gold salts in the treatment of asthma must be regarded as investigational.

Antihistamines

The first-generation antihistamines—diphenhydramine (Benadryl) and chlorpheniramine (Chlortrimeton)—have long been regarded as contraindicated in asthmatics. This prohibition has stemmed from the drying effect older antihistamines have on lung secretions and the greater potential for "plugging" of the bronchial tubes in asthmatic attacks.

The second-generation agents—loratadine (Claritin), desloratadine (Clarinex), cetirizine (Zyrtec), and fexofenadine (Allegra)—have a variety of anti-inflammatory properties that include a decrease in mast cell release of asthma mediators. These effects are mild, however, so that the benefit in asthma control may be negligible. The combination of a second-generation antihistamine with an anti-leukotriene, however, may augment these effects.

Azelastine. Azelastine is an antihistamine that has undergone trials in patients with bronchial asthma in Japan and other countries. Despite early positive results no significant benefit has been proven in large numbers of patients. One adverse effect is drowsiness. This drug is available in the United States as a nasal spray (Astelin) for relief of allergic rhinitis.

Ketotifen. Another antihistamine, ketotifen, has been available for use in Europe for bronchial asthma. To date, studies do not demonstrate a significant beneficial effect. This agent may also cause drowsiness. There are no plans to introduce this drug in the United States.

Gammaglobulin

Gammaglobulin is a protein substance that normally circulates in the blood to combat infection. A small number of severely asthmatic patients have been treated with intravenous infusions of gammaglobulin. Selected patients who received gammaglobulin have been able to reduce their steroid requirements. However, this treatment should be considered investigational since only a small number of patients have undergone this form of therapy.

It should be noted that gammaglobulin is often administered to patients who are born with a deficiency of this important substance. Often these patients experience frequent infections that may affect the sinuses and bronchial tubes. Some of these patients also have bronchial asthma, and treatment of the gammaglobulin deficiency may actually result in improvement of the asthmatic condition. This "replacement therapy" differs from the investigational use of gammaglobulin in bronchial asthma just noted.

Are Asthma Medications Addictive?

Many patients fear they will become addicted to their asthma medications and be unable to stop their use. This fear may partly be due to dependence on medication for the relief of symptoms and attacks and may explain why some patients do not take their medications.

There is no evidence of the development of addiction to asthma medications. When good control of asthma is achieved, it is often possible to reduce or discontinue medication that is no longer needed. However, good control must come first since withdrawal of medication may result in increased frequency of attacks.

Adrenal Insufficiency

In the case of systemic corticosteroids, the management of reduction and withdrawal of these agents must be closely supervised in view of possible adrenal insufficiency. Patients with severe asthma may become "steroid dependent" for control of their disease but that does not represent an addiction to medication.

Are There Delayed Effects of Asthma Medications?

Patients may be concerned whether long-term use of asthma drugs will have serious adverse effects, another reason why patients may reduce or eliminate medications on their own.

Long-term use in adults of the β-agonists, theophylline, cromolyn sodium, ipratropium bromide, nedocromil, anti-leukotrienes, and inhaled corticosteroids has not shown any evidence of delayed adverse effects. In children, low- to medium-dose inhaled corticosteroids have not shown adverse effects on growth and bone development. High-dose inhaled corticosteroids may still be necessary when the risk of severe, uncontrolled asthma outweighs the possible detrimental effects on bone growth.

Oral Corticosteroids

In both children and adults, long-term effects of the oral corticosteroids must be anticipated. These side effects have been described and must be weighed against the dangers of uncontrolled asthma. Once systemic steroids are required, there should be frequent review of their necessity with the goal of reducing dosage or withdrawal if possible. Alternate-day administration should always be considered if patients must remain on oral corticosteroids.

How Should Asthma Drugs Be Used?

In this chapter specific asthma medications have been discussed. As the number of medications and their effectiveness increase, confusion has also increased as to how these medications should be taken. Patients are often given several different medications and may find it difficult to use them all. Many patients complain they are "overmedicated" and stop medications on their own. Chapter 5 provides a strategy for using asthma medications effectively.

5

Strategy for
Medication Treatment

Treating asthma requires a step-by-step approach in order to provide the correct medication. In general, therapy is initiated at a higher level to establish prompt control and is then "stepped down" to reduce the risk of adverse effects of medication. This "step therapy" also ensures that medication will be given in the proper dosage and that unnecessary medication will not be given. To prescribe the correct asthma medication, a physician must grade patients according to the severity of their condition. This chapter defines asthma in terms of its severity and proposes a strategy for treatment based on degree of severity.

Adult Asthma: Mild, Moderate, and Severe

The National Institutes of Health (NIH) has categorized asthma as "mild intermittent," "mild persistent," "moderate persistent," and "severe persistent." Mild intermittent asthma is defined as a condition in which attacks do not occur more than twice a week and never during sleep. Between attacks, peak flow rates are maintained at more than 80 percent of normal. Mild persistent asthmatics have symptoms more than twice a week but less than once a day. Their peak flows are greater than 80 percent of normal. Moderate persistent asthmatics have daily symptoms and one nocturnal attack per week. Their peak flows are between 60 percent and 80 percent of normal. Severe persistent asthmatics have continuous symptoms. They require regular bronchodilator use, often need oral corticosteroid courses, have been hospitalized for severe attacks usually with assisted respiration, and often have night attacks. Peak flow measurements are less than 60 percent of normal. Steroid-dependent asthmatics form a subgroup of these severe patients. These patients are never without oral corticosteroids due to continuous symptoms.

Use Severity Definitions Cautiously

These severity definitions are helpful but should not be employed rigidly. It should be emphasized that patients at any level may experience severe, life-threatening asthmatic attacks. These severe attacks may occur suddenly after long symptom-free periods with normal lung function. Patients with allergic or extrinsic asthma may only be symptomatic during certain seasons depending on the amount of pollen to which they are exposed. Some allergic patients experience symptoms only when exposed to certain allergens such as cat dander; others may display symptoms only during an upper respiratory tract infection such as a sore throat or sinus infection. A few patients will be symptomatic only after exercise. All these patients could also be defined as mild asthmatics even though their attacks may sometimes be severe. To be sure, asthma severity varies from patient to patient and strict definitions are not easily applied.

Strategy for Treatment: Step Therapy

All patients should have a strategy for treatment that they have discussed and agreed to after consulting with their physicians. It is best that these instructions be in writing for easy reference and that close communication (aided by peak flow measurements) be maintained with the physician. Often the details of a "strategy" will be revised. No treatment plan should ever be regarded as final, since there are frequent variations in asthma as well as new medications that become available. Treatment is best given in a "step-by-step" fashion, avoiding simultaneous administration of several new agents, so the physician and patient can more accurately determine what treatment is most effective.

Treatment Goals

Treatment goals for bronchial asthma are maintaining a normal lifestyle, including vigorous exercise; reversing bronchial narrowing, inflammation, and irritability, thereby sustaining "normal" lung function; and avoiding adverse medication effects. Symptoms such as shortness of breath, wheezing, and coughing should be minimal. Whenever medication side effects such as those encountered with long-term oral corticosteroids outweigh benefits, the medication program must be revised.

Treatment Strategy: Mild Asthma

Mild intermittent asthma can often be treated with infrequent use of a β_2-adrenergic agonist delivered by metered-dose inhaler (MDI). The β-agonist would be used "as needed," not regularly. Short-acting agents are preferred because of their more rapid onset.

Patients with mild persistent asthma require the addition of an anti-inflammatory agent, which is used on a regular basis. The preferred agent is an inhaled corticosteroid (in low doses). An anti-leukotriene, cromolyn, and nedocromil are alternatives. Cromolyn and nedocromil may be helpful in cough asthma where blockage of bronchial nerve reflexes often reduces symptoms.

It should be noted that one study has suggested that mild persistent asthmatics may not require regular use of an inhaled steroid. Patients in this study were treated with inhaled or oral corticosteroids on an "as-needed basis." Further studies will be needed to confirm these results.

Treatment Strategy: Moderate Asthma

Patients with moderate persistent asthma require higher doses of topical corticosteroids and the addition of a long-acting inhaled β_2-agonist (salmeterol or formoterol). This medication is administered every twelve hours on a regular basis. Fixed-combination inhalers that include a corticosteroid and long-acting β_2-agonist are available (Advair Diskus). Patients with moderate persistent asthma may continue to use a short-acting β_2-agonist spray when symptoms break through. This has been appropriately termed "rescue" medication. Adding a long-acting β_2-agonist, however, frequently results in a reduction in the use of the short-acting agent. In view of the detrimental effects of overuse of β-agonists, this reduction is highly beneficial. Due to the slow onset of action, it must be emphasized that the long-acting β-agonist must not be used for relief of acute asthmatic attacks.

Alternative agents for these patients include sustained-release β_2-agonist tablets, theophylline, and the anti-leukotrienes.

The Next Step in Moderate Asthma. Patients in the moderate group who are still symptomatic with reduced activity and flow rates despite the combination of a long-acting β_2-adrenergic agonist and medium doses of an inhaled corticosteroid will require additional second-line therapy. For bronchodilatation, adding an oral preparation of the β-agonist theophylline and/or ipratropium bromide may be helpful. Those with nocturnal symptoms may respond to evening administration of a long-acting β_2-agonist or theophylline. If attacks continue to be frequent, a trial of an additional anti-inflammatory agent is the next step. An anti-leukotriene or cromolyn or nedocromil may be added. It should be emphasized again that the decision to start or stop medications should be based on objective findings (spirometry or peak flow readings) in addition to the patient's symptoms and frequency of attacks.

Patients with moderate asthma with frequent exacerbations despite the medications just described often require courses of oral corticosteroids. It is always helpful before starting oral corticosteroids to review the correct use of MDI sprays as well as to emphasize the use and benefit of a spacer. Discussions between patient and physician must be frequent in this group to reiterate individual goals of treatment and to discuss the potential side effects of oral corticosteroids. Often it will become clear that a medication (usually inhaled corticosteroid) has not been used due to fear of dependency or side effects. It has been estimated that one-third to one-half of these patients do not adhere to their asthma therapy. When medication questions are answered satisfactorily, resumption of therapy may avoid the use of oral steroids and their side effects.

Patients who are compliant with their medications and have documented moderate to severe allergic or extrinsic asthma should be considered for treatment with omalizumab (Xolair).

Treatment Strategy: Severe Asthma

In the patient with severe persistent asthma, a home nebulizer should be considered. This device may be used to deliver not only a β_2-adrenergic agonist but also inhaled corticosteroid (Pulmicort Respules), cromolyn sodium, and ipratropium bromide. This combined aerosol therapy may be extremely helpful in certain patients. A nebulizer may not prove more advantageous than medication delivered by MDI for every patient.

Patients with severe persistent asthma require high doses of inhaled corticosteroids, long-acting β_2-agonist, theophylline, and frequent courses of oral corticosteroid. Maintenance oral steroid may also be necessary. This should always be given in the smallest dose that is effective and only after a trial of alternate-day therapy. The addition of an anti-leukotriene may permit a reduction in the daily steroid dosage. This reduction must be done carefully with monitoring for the development of adrenal insufficiency. Patients with documented severe allergic asthma should be treated with omalizumab (Xolair). Those patients with severe nonallergic or intrinsic asthma should be considered candidates for trials of etanercept (Enbrel) or other third-line agents, such as methotrexate. Table 5.1 shows the step-by-step treatment strategy for mild, moderate, and severe asthma.

The Peak Flow Meter and the Acute Attack

As outlined in Chapter 3, peak flow meter readings may be used to direct the management of an acute asthmatic attack. The patient's

Table 5.1   Step-By-Step Strategy for Treatment of Asthma in Adults and Children Older than Five Years of Age

Mild Intermittent Asthma

Inhaled β₂-agonist as needed

Mild Persistent Asthma

Add an anti-inflammatory agent:

Preferred: Low-dose inhaled corticosteroid

Alternatives: Anti-leukotriene, cromolyn, nedocromil, theophylline

Moderate Persistent Asthma

Add a long-acting inhaled β₂-agonist every twelve hours

Alternatives: Increase inhaled corticosteroid to medium dose or add anti-leukotriene or theophylline to low-dose steroid

Severe Persistent Asthma

Use high-dose inhaled corticosteroid, long-acting inhaled β₂-agonist, anti-leukotriene, theophylline

Add oral corticosteroids for exacerbations in tapering dosages

Add omalizumab in allergic patients with elevated IgE and positive allergy tests

strategy for treatment should include peak flow meter readings, and the patient and physician should design a plan of treatment based largely on peak flow measurements. Once the patient has obtained a "personal best" value, changes in this "normal" reading can be used to direct therapy. Changes in peak flow of 25 percent, 50 percent, and 75 percent are useful guidelines for assessing the severity of an attack and how the patient should respond. To avoid serious episodes, treatment should be initiated at the earliest indication of an attack (25 percent decrease in peak flow).

Oral corticosteroids should be used for significant drops in flow (50 percent decrease). Emergency medical attention should be given for severe decreases (75 percent drop in peak flow). Table 5.2 is an example of a plan of action for acute asthmatic attacks.

Table 5.2   Plan of Treatment for Acute Attacks Based on Peak Flow Measurements

Measure peak flow twice a day.

Obtain "personal best" value.

If Peak Flow Falls by 25 Percent

Use β_2-agonist for immediate relief.

If improvement is not maintained, increase inhaled steroid.

If Peak Flow Falls by 50 Percent

Use β_2-agonist for immediate relief.

Begin course of oral corticosteroid.

Inform physician.

If Peak Flow Falls by 75 Percent

Use β_2-agonist for immediate relief.

Begin oral corticosteroid and seek medical attention.

The National Asthma Education and Prevention Program

The National Heart, Lung, and Blood Institute (NHLB) and its National Asthma Education and Prevention Program (NAEPP) convened a panel of experts on the management of asthma that has released a series of comprehensive reports ("Guidelines for the Diagnosis and Management of Asthma") since 1991. This excellent resource has included a suggestion for a "traffic light system" that would allow patients to easily remember how to manage their asthma. This green-yellow-red zone system has been adopted by many physicians and has been included in many peak flow meter designs.

The Green Zone

As defined by the NAEPP, the green zone is a safe area in which the asthma patient experiences few or no symptoms. Peak flow measurements are 80 percent to 100 percent of a patient's predicted normal value or personal best with no more than a 20 percent swing in values. Medications are individualized for each patient, whether they are mild, moderate, or severe asthmatics.

The Yellow Zone

The yellow zone, as outlined by the NAEPP, signals "caution." The patient has peak flows that are 50 percent to 80 percent of his or her predicted normal or personal best and/or asthma symptoms that may include nocturnal attacks, coughing, wheezing, decreased activity, and chest tightness. This "zone" indicates that medications should be adjusted according to the management plan suggested by the physician. Patients who make frequent visits to the yellow zone should have their maintenance medications reviewed and adjusted.

The Red Zone

The red zone signals a "medical alert." Peak flows are below 50 percent of the predicted value or personal best, and asthma symptoms are frequent, including at rest. The patient's management plan should immediately be put into place for this degree of attack, as previously described. Typically, this calls for immediate use of a β-agonist and introduction of oral corticosteroids. Patients who do not respond require immediate medical attention, usually an emergency room visit. Patients who fall into the red zone should certainly have their maintenance asthma programs reviewed and adjusted.

Should This Terminology Be Used?

The simple terminology suggested by the NAEPP is helpful to patients in managing their asthma. For anyone familiar with traffic signals, it is certainly easy to remember. Peak flow meters are usually green-yellow-red coded. Remember, however, that treatment decisions should be based on prior consultation with the physician and the patient's record of personal best flows and not by color zones alone. Each patient should have green, yellow, and red zones defined with written guidelines for treatment decisions.

Childhood Asthma

Chronic asthma is the most frequent long-term children's disease. Acute asthmatic attacks usually occur at the time of a cough or cold caused by a viral infection. In evaluating the childhood asthmatic the physician must rely more on the patient's history and physical findings since measurements of pulmonary function may be difficult to obtain. This is particularly true for children under five years of age. Children older than five are generally able to provide peak flow measurements. The diagnosis of asthma may be particularly difficult since wheezing in children is most often due to colds rather than asthma.

What Should a Parent Look For?

In the child's history the physician will ask for evidence of cough and wheezing. Wheezing is usually heard when the child breathes out. Coughing may be prolonged without a cold and is often worse at night. Changes in a child's activity may reflect shortness of breath, especially if there is difficulty during exercise. Parents should take note if their children no longer wish to play physical games they used to enjoy or take other exercise. Awakening at night may reflect nocturnal asthma. As in adults, the presence of nasal symptoms (drip, sneezing, and congestion) may signal an allergy and increase the likelihood of asthma. A strong family history of allergy or asthma may help identify the childhood asthmatic.

What Does the Physical Examination Show?

The physical examination of an asthmatic child does not greatly differ from that performed on the adult. Once again, the presence of wheezing does not confirm the diagnosis and may occur with respiratory infections or colds. In a child there is also a greater incidence of foreign body aspiration, which may produce wheezing and mimic asthma. Cystic fibrosis must be considered in a child with cough, sputum production, and wheezing. As in the adult patient, wheezing may be absent or intermittent.

Asthma in Infants

Asthma may occur in infants. More than half of childhood patients developed their first symptoms before age two. The most common source of asthma in children six months of age or younger is viral infection. This is often viral bronchitis or pneumonia. Indications of asthma in this age group may be a change in the child's cry or ability to feed or suckle. Children breathe rapidly but an increase in this rate or change in skin color due to a lack of oxygen, called cyanosis, may be significant indicators of asthma. Since the physician is unable to rely on measurements of airflow to determine the severity of asthma in this young age group, measurement of blood oxygen is often necessary.

What Are the Common Triggers?

Childhood asthma is usually triggered by colds. In allergic children, exposure to allergens such as pollen, dust, animal dander, mold, and dust mites may precipitate attacks. Food allergies, such as an allergy to nuts, are much more common in childhood asthmatics than in adults. Cigarette or pipe smoke as well as pollution and dust produce irritation that may also trigger asthmatic attacks. Children exposed to secondhand smoke have been found to develop greater numbers of respiratory infections, the primary asthma trigger. Parents are strongly encouraged to quit smoking.

Treatment Strategy: Mild Childhood Asthma

In mild intermittent childhood asthma the initial treatment is use of the β_2-adrenergic agonist. Due to the difficulty younger patients (under age five) have using MDIs, there must be increased reliance on nebulized medication and oral preparations (chewable tablets, granules, or elixirs). Use of an MDI with a spacer and face mask attachment may be particularly helpful in young patients to ensure better delivery of aerosol medication. As with adult patients there is a greater chance of side effects (nervousness or tremor) in a child receiving oral medication.

Children with mild persistent asthma should add an anti-inflammatory agent in the form of an inhaled corticosteroid. This may be given with a nebulizer (Pulmicort Respules), DPI (Pulmicort Turbuhaler, Flovent Rotadisk) or an MDI with a spacer with or without a face mask. Mometasone (Asmanex) is currently approved for teenagers age twelve or older.

Alternative agents are cromolyn, which is available for nebulizer use or as an MDI; nedocromil, approved for children aged six months and older; or an anti-leukotriene. Studies comparing the inhaled corticosteroids and these alternative agents as well as theophylline have revealed a clear superiority of the inhaled corticosteroid in improving asthma outcomes.

Low to medium dosages of inhaled corticosteroids in children up to six years of age are considered safe with the benefits of asthma control greatly exceeding the small risk of side effects on growth and adrenal function. Children followed for more than ten years on these dosages were found to reach their final predicted height. Long-term studies have not shown any effect on bone density or the incidence of cataracts or glaucoma. The side effects of using higher dosages of inhaled corticosteroids in children should be weighed against the effects of uncontrolled asthma.

Treatment Strategy: Moderate Childhood Asthma

Children with moderate persistent asthma experience daily symptoms and have more than two attacks each week. These patients require the addition of a long-acting β_2-agonist such as salmeterol (age four and older) or formoterol (age five and older) given every twelve hours. These agents are also approved for the prevention of exercise-induced asthma in children. Children with primarily nocturnal symptoms may use one inhalation nightly. If asthma symptoms persist, a higher dosage of the inhaled corticosteroid may be necessary and an anti-leukotriene or theophylline may be added.

Theophylline. Theophylline is a second-line agent for use in uncontrolled childhood asthma. Unfortunate side effects such as nervousness, however, limit its usefulness. Recent studies have raised the question of a learning disability that may be attributed to theophylline. Additional adverse effects are stomach upset and headache. As in adults, blood levels must be monitored to ensure an effective therapeutic level.

Anticholinergic Agents. The anticholinergic agent ipratropium bromide may be used in children aged five and older as a second- or third-line agent. Since most childhood asthmatics are allergic, it is not likely that this agent would provide significant broncho-dilatation. It is available in a nebulizer form as well as an MDI. There is no available information on the use of tiotropium bromide in children.

Treatment Strategy: Severe Childhood Asthma

Severe childhood asthmatics require high-dose inhaled corticosteroids, long-acting β_2-agonists, and the addition of oral corticosteroids. These patients continue to have several attacks a week and reduced airflows despite maximal therapy. The adverse effects of oral corticosteroids are similar to those of adults but are more significant in regard to growth and bone development in the youngest patients. Alternate-day therapy should be attempted for patients who require maintenance steroid therapy due to severe disease. Teenagers age twelve or older with severe allergic asthma are good candidates for treatment with omalizumab (Xolair).

Table 5.3 shows the step-by-step treatment strategy for children under age five.

When Do I Call the Doctor?

In older children the use of a peak flow meter provides a useful tool for home monitoring of your child's asthma. Similar to adults, drops in peak flow of 25 percent or more should be reported to your pediatrician and a contingency plan should be in place. Electronic peak flow meters are available that permit the downloading

Table 5.3 *Step-By-Step Strategy for Treatment of Asthma in Infants and Children Under Five Years of Age*

Mild Intermittent Asthma

Use inhaled β_2-agonist as needed.

Mild Persistent Asthma

Add an anti-inflammatory agent:

Preferred: Low-dose inhaled corticosteroid (with nebulizer or MDI with face mask or DPI)

Alternatives: Anti-leukotriene or cromolyn (with nebulizer or MDI with face mask)

Moderate Persistent Asthma

Add a long-acting inhaled β_2-agonist every twelve hours.

Alternatives: Increase inhaled corticosteroid to medium dose or add anti-leukotriene or theophylline to low-dose steroid.

Severe Persistent Asthma

Use high-dose inhaled corticosteroid, long-acting inhaled β_2-agonist, anti-leukotriene, theophylline.

Add oral corticosteroids for exacerbations in tapering dosages.

of peak flows directly to your physician's office. For a sample plan of action for acute asthma attacks, see Table 5.2.

In very young children, any trouble in breathing or a change in skin color to white or blue (especially of the lips and fingernails) should be reported to your doctor. You should also report when your child's regular asthma medication does not appear to work.

Managing Asthma in the Elderly

Asthma may occur at any age. One of my earliest patients was a woman who developed allergy and asthma at age eighty-four. She had seen several other physicians who had rejected the possibility that someone of her age might develop asthma and told her instead that she had emphysema ("because I was old"). Her laboratory evaluation revealed several positive allergy tests ("I was never allergic before and now I am sneezing all the time"), and her pulmonary function tests confirmed asthma. She improved markedly with the appropriate treatment for moderate persistent asthma and continues to do well.

In some older patients, asthma may also recur after a long hiatus. Former or current smokers may have components of both asthma and chronic obstructive pulmonary disease (COPD), making the diagnosis and treatment of asthma in the elderly particularly challenging.

Asthma or COPD?

It is important for the physician to distinguish between asthma and COPD for several reasons. Asthma has a more favorable natural course and better chance of responding to treatment. The use of medication in these two illnesses is also different. Inhaled corticosteroids are more effective in asthma, and anti-cholinergic bronchodilators are more helpful in COPD patients.

When distinguishing asthma from COPD in an elderly patient, the physician must first consider whether there is a history of smoking or exposure to secondhand smoke. The physical examination may not be helpful since wheezing is common in both entities. Pulmonary function testing, however, should provide valuable diagnostic evidence. Individuals with asthma experience a marked response to bronchodilator medication whereas COPD patients have a much less pronounced response. In addition, the diffusion capacity (see Chapter 2) is normal in asthmatics but significantly reduced in COPD patients.

Pulmonary function testing, however, may fail to make the distinction between asthma and COPD in asthmatic patients with chronically constricted airways. These patients may fail to improve after bronchodilator, often leading to a misdiagnosis of COPD. In these patients, a course of oral corticosteroids may be necessary to "unmask" the diagnosis of asthma by first reducing airway swelling and inflammation.

A chest CAT scan may also be diagnostic in many patients since it may directly visualize areas of emphysema or bronchitis. These changes may not be seen on a plain chest x-ray. In both asthmatics and COPD patients, the lungs may appear larger than normal, or "hyperinflated," on x-ray due to slow emptying of air through narrowed airways.

Are the Treatment Goals Different for the Elderly?

The goal of asthma treatment is to achieve a normal lifestyle. This includes obtaining normal lung function. In the elderly patient these goals may be more difficult to achieve since chronic asthma may produce severely reduced breathing capacity and constricted airways. These patients often restrict their activities due to shortness of breath and may require a rehabilitation program to improve their quality of life.

Education

Elderly patients may require additional education on the proper use of medication. Many of my elderly patients have had difficulty using an MDI due to arthritis or reduced hand strength. In these patients, a nebulizer or dry powder inhaler proved to be more suitable. Education may also be needed for family members or in-home caregivers to ensure compliance with treatment.

Peak Flows

The use of a peak flow meter may also be difficult for many elderly patients. In these individuals close monitoring of symptoms using a diary may prove useful. Important symptoms to record include awakenings during the night or early morning with wheezing or cough, more frequent cough, increased use of the "rescue" inhaler, and decreased exercise tolerance. The diary entries can be discussed with the physician at office visits or by phone.

Environmental Triggers

In elderly asthmatics, respiratory infections appear to play a greater role in triggering attacks than inhaled allergens. Vaccination with influenza (annually) and pneumococcal vaccine (every five to seven years) is especially important in this population. Smoking and exposure to secondhand smoke must be avoided. In the allergic individual, allergy control measures should be instituted. (See Chapter 6.)

Medications

The stepwise approach outlined previously should be followed in all patients with asthma. Older patients, however, have an increased risk of adverse effects, which may limit the choice, dosage, and frequency of medications. In addition, these patients often take multiple medications for a variety of conditions, increasing the risk of drug interactions.

Inhaled Corticosteroids. A number of adverse effects of inhaled corticosteroids may be noted in the elderly, especially with high doses. These include thinning and bruising of the skin, loss of bone mineral content, and accelerated osteoporosis. Bone density tests are indicated for these patients, and measures to reduce the risk of osteoporosis should be carefully followed.

Systemic Corticosteroids. Corticosteroids taken by mouth or by injection pose an even greater risk of adverse effects in the elderly population because these medications break down slower in these patients. These additional effects include fluid retention, electrolyte imbalance, bone fractures, depression, stomach ulcers, worsening glaucoma, and cataracts. As in all individuals with asthma, the dosage of systemic corticosteroids should be reduced as soon as possible.

Theophylline. Older patients may not tolerate theophylline due to an increased susceptibility to adverse side effects, which include nausea, cardiac arrhythmias, and insomnia. A number of medications are also known to interact with theophylline, requiring an adjustment in dosage. In elderly patients, theophylline blood levels should be followed closely with a target range of 8 to 12 mg/mL.

Beta-Agonists. B-agonists may produce more frequent adverse effects in the elderly population. These include cardiac arrhythmias, tremors, and reduction in potassium levels. Elderly patients may also have preexisting heart disease, further increasing the risk of an adverse effect. Oral preparations of β-agonists should be avoided due to possible tremors as well as increased heart rate. Long-acting β_2-agonists also commonly produce tremors and rapid heart rate in this population and may not be tolerated. Patients who develop adverse effects due to β-agonists may be treated with an anti-cholinergic bronchodilator. (See Chapter 4.)

Medications That May Adversely Affect Asthma

Older patients commonly have coexisting medical conditions (cardiovascular disease, glaucoma, and arthritis, for example) that require medications that may adversely affect asthma.

Beta-Blockers. A commonly prescribed group of medications, beta-blockers may produce severe, life-threatening asthmatic attacks. These medications are widely prescribed for multiple illnesses, including hypertension, cardiac arrhythmia, angina pectoris, glaucoma, and migraine.

When active or stimulated, the beta-receptors located in the lung (called beta-2 receptors) produce relaxation of the muscle surrounding the bronchial tubes, which widens the bronchial passage (bronchodilatation). If these receptors are blocked from receiving nerve input, the reverse effect (bronchoconstriction) results. This may have devastating effects on patients with underlying bronchial asthma.

Beta-receptors are present in other organ systems such as the heart and circulation; these are referred to as beta-1 receptors. Beta-blockers that affect beta-1 receptors more than beta-2 receptors are termed "selective." These medications vary in potency and duration. A number of the selective beta-blockers produce less blockade of lung receptors, but there is still significant risk for exacerbating bronchial asthma. As a rule, all beta-blockers should be avoided by asthma patients. If an asthma patient must take a beta-blocker, a selective agent should be used.

Don't Forget Eyedrops! Beta-blockers in the form of eyedrops are commonly used to treat glaucoma. Medication may be absorbed from the eye and delivered into the general blood circulation before reaching the bronchial tubes. Patients with bronchial asthma have suffered asthmatic attacks from beta-blockers introduced into the eye for treating glaucoma. Selective beta-blockers have been developed for glaucoma but may also produce bronchoconstriction. All patients with bronchial asthma should inform their ophthalmologists of their lung condition before treatment for glaucoma is initiated. In severe glaucoma cases where a beta-blocker is felt to be necessary, a selective agent should be used and the patient's airflows closely monitored.

Diuretics. Older patients frequently require diuretics ("water pills") for high blood pressure or heart failure. When diuretics that do not spare potassium are combined with β-agonists, a drop in potassium and magnesium levels may result. This electrolyte imbalance may produce heart arrhythmias, particularly in patients receiving a heart medication known as digitalis. Patients should be monitored closely with blood levels, and supplements should be given when an imbalance occurs.

Angiotensin-Converting Enzyme Inhibitors. Elderly patients frequently are given angiotensin-converting enzyme (ACE) inhibitors for high blood pressure. These agents may produce chronic cough. Individuals with asthma have a greater frequency of this side effect. The withdrawal of the ACE inhibitor should eliminate the cough.

Nonsteroidal Anti-Inflammatory Drugs. Older patients frequently develop arthritis and may be treated with aspirin and nonsteroidal anti-inflammatory drugs. These agents may cause sudden and severe asthmatic attacks. (See Chapter 11.)

Putting Your Strategy to Work

In this chapter asthma has been defined as mild, moderate, and severe, with specific treatment strategies proposed for each category. A system based on traffic signal colors is in wide use, but whatever strategy is used for the treatment of asthma, its success depends on a working partnership between patient and physician. Up to this point the physician has directed treatment and provided guidelines. Chapter 6 discusses the patient's role in treatment.

6

How to Participate in Managing Your Asthma

FOR AN ASTHMA treatment strategy to succeed, the patient must be an active participant. Patients who take an active role in their care have better control over their disease. The health benefits from patient participation can be applied to any illness but seems particularly true in diseases such as asthma and diabetes. Patients who participate in their own care are better educated in regard to their illness and can communicate well with their physicians. These characteristics are extremely important in managing bronchial asthma. This chapter discusses the steps patients can take to become active participants in their care, and specific suggestions are offered regarding diet, stress, and work.

Self-Monitoring and Education

In managing bronchial asthma a patient can play an active role in decision making by closely monitoring airflows with a home peak flow meter, as described in Chapter 3. From the record of the peak flows a physician can judge the effectiveness of treatment, evaluate the patient's response to new drugs, pinpoint adverse environmental influences at home and work, and determine the need for emergency management. Peak flows may also be used for special situations such as before and after exercise to determine a patient's response to various asthma triggers.

Your physician should be your primary source of information about asthma. Limits on time may prevent discussion of all important issues on an initial visit, so make a list of topics you want to discuss so you can raise these issues during follow-up visits. Ask your doctor about recommended reading to further your education. Before leaving the physician's office you should have been taught the correct use of a metered-dose inhaler (MDI), peak flow meter, and spacer, if they are prescribed. Videotapes of proper inhalation techniques for using MDIs are available. Written instructions on the use of your medications should be given to you. Ask lots of questions. Two excellent questions are: "What are the side effects I should be aware of?" "Are there any drug interactions with my other medicines?"

At home, keep a record of your doctor's office visits and appointments. A diary of your peak flow measurements should also be maintained. Mark your calendar when you start using an MDI so you can mark ahead the date when it should be refilled. Always carry a list of your medications with you as well as a fresh bronchodilator spray for emergency use. If you travel, carry a set of your prescriptions in case your medication is mislaid. Research the climate you will be traveling to as well as important aspects of the locale such as local allergens or the altitude. Ask your physician about the effects of altitude on your condition and whether you should have prescriptions for emergency medications such as antibiotics or corticosteroids.

Is Your Asthma Under Control?

A recent poll asked several thousand adults with asthma if they thought their asthma was under control. Eighty-eighty percent said yes, but almost half of these individuals also reported that symptoms disturbed their sleep and stopped them from exercising. These symptoms actually indicate a lack of control. It is clear that people with asthma tend to think they have much better control over their conditions than they actually do. This may also be a misconception of parents of children with asthma. They may assume that their child doesn't like sports when in fact the child may develop short-ness of breath while exercising and stop competing.

A simple test of your asthma "control" is whether you have asthma symptoms more than twice a week during the daytime or more than two nights a month. If you do, then your asthma is not adequately controlled and you should bring this to the attention of your physician. You may also take the American Lung Association's Asthma Control Test™ on the Internet (see the Appendix) and obtain an "asthma score." Uncontrolled asthma produces chronic inflammation and swelling ("remodeling") of the bronchial tubes, which may become permanent if left untreated.

Choosing Your Asthma Physician

Many types of physicians administer treatment to patients with bronchial asthma. Family physicians, pediatricians, internists, allergists, and pulmonologists are all involved in treatment of patients with asthma. Excellent care may be provided by any of these types of physicians who are well trained and experienced in treatment of asthma. An asthma specialist is often a physician who has specialty training in asthma as well as other chest diseases, such as a pulmonologist. Patients with unstable asthma or disease that is unresponsive to treatment should certainly be seen by an asthma specialist who can work in concert with the primary physician. Even patients with mild disease may benefit from a specialist's review of their diagnosis and treatment. Patients with asthma should undergo an allergy evaluation, which may be administered under the direction of an allergist.

Many factors enter into your choice of a physician in addition to training and expertise. It should be apparent to each patient if the "chemistry is right" and that a good rapport has been established with a physician. How the physician responds to questions and listens to concerns about chronic disease, fears of medication effects, and descriptions of side effects should make it clear if the right choice of a physician has been made. Choose a caring, empathic physician since close communication between patient and physician is likely to improve the outcome of treatment. Other important considerations are availability and how emergency calls are handled, as well as access to facilities for evaluation and treatment. Finally, the patient must feel that a partnership has been established with the physician for achieving the best possible care.

Reducing Allergens at Home and Work

The patient can take an active role in managing the environment at home and in the office. In allergic patients, avoiding offending allergen(s) may drastically reduce the frequency of asthmatic attacks. Allergens can be identified through a history of reaction and skin or blood testing. Common allergens are dust mites, mold spores, animal dander, and plant pollens. Insects such as the cockroach may also produce allergens that precipitate attacks. Specific allergens may be identified through testing of samples taken from the home. Table 6.1 includes specific allergy-proofing tips for home and office.

Dust Mites

Dust mites may play a significant role in many asthmatic attacks. These extremely small insects depend on moisture for survival and live on human skin dander. They have been found in abundant quantities in mattresses, pillows, clothes, bed coverings, carpets, towels, and even stuffed animals. In the home, the highest concentrations have been found in the bedroom. It is the feces of the dust mite that produces an allergic reaction. Because these droppings are airborne when dust is disturbed, they can be inhaled and cause allergic reactions. The particles are large enough to be trapped, however, and the patient can significantly reduce the number of dust mites through specific measures.

Prevention measures include trapping dust mites by using a zippered mattress and pillow cover. Sheets and bed covers should be washed weekly in hot water. Carpeting should be removed wherever possible, and any remaining carpeting treated with a chemical agent (acaracide) such as benzyl benzoate (Acarosan) or tannic acid that kills mites. (See Figure 6.1.) For more informa-

Table 6.1   Tips for Allergy-Proofing Your Home or Office

To Reduce Dust Mites

Remove carpets, rugs, and upholstered furniture.

Encase mattresses, pillows, and box springs in zippered covers.

Wash sheets and bedding in hot water weekly.

Wash stuffed animals.

Use a HEPA air filter.

To Reduce Mold

Keep humidity levels at 30 percent to 50 percent with a dehumidifier.

Use a mold remover spray on bathroom and basement walls, windowsills, air conditioners, humidifiers, and plant soil.

Remove carpeting over concrete floors.

Use a HEPA air filter.

To Reduce Indoor Pollution

Ban smoking from your home.

Avoid gas and wood stoves and fireplaces.

Avoid cooking odors with an exhaust fan; avoid paint fumes.

Use an air conditioner, HEPA filter to keep out pollens, particulates, and fumes.

tion on obtaining these materials, see the Appendix. Vacuuming is important and should be done once a week, preferably not by the asthma patient. If you must vacuum yourself, use a dust mask and a vacuum cleaner with high-density paper bags and filtration as well as a High Efficiency Particulate Air (HEPA) filter. Indoor humidity levels should be reduced to less than 50 percent with a dehumidifier.

Air Filters. An air filter may be helpful in reducing allergen levels for the dust mite as well as other offending substances. Air filters may be mechanical or electrical. One of the best mechanical types incorporates a HEPA filter. These come in various sizes according to the volume of the room (amount of air) that has to be filtered and circulated. Know the dimensions of the room in which the air

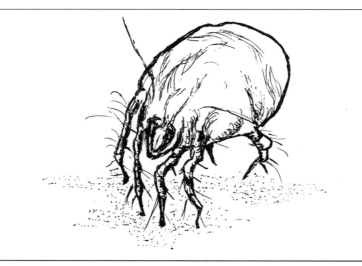

Figure 6.1 Dust mite

filter will be placed before you purchase one. Electrical and HEPA filters can also be placed in a central forced air system in the home. The HEPA units require periodic replacement of filters and the electrical units require regular cleaning.

One example of an electrical filter is the electrostatic precipitator, which traps particles on oppositely charged plates and is often referred to as an "ionizing air filter." Recent testing has revealed that some ionizing models produce significant amounts of ozone. Ozone is present in the upper atmosphere where it acts as a shield against ultraviolet rays. When ozone is present at ground level it is an irritant that can aggravate asthma and worsen lung function. In addition, research suggests that ozone interacts with the terpenes in lemon- and pine-scented cleaning products and air fresheners, creating formaldehyde and other irritants. These by-products can be absorbed by beds and carpets and be released over long periods of time. Ultrafine particles may also be released by this interaction, which can penetrate deep into lungs. Electrical filters require more frequent cleaning than mechanical types. Some of the ionizing filters are now equipped with a catalyst that reduces the amount of ozone released.

Tests of performance of both HEPA and electrical air filters are available through *Consumer Reports* and other independent organizations. Review of these test results is recommended before purchasing any unit. Overall, based on the data revealing ozone production by ionizing air filters, a HEPA unit is preferred as an air cleaner.

Molds

Molds are fungi that grow well in warm and moist environments. (See Figure 6.2.) They are frequently found in the bathroom, kitchen, and basement of homes. Airborne mold spores are the allergens that can produce asthmatic attacks in sensitive individuals. Many steps can be taken to reduce mold spores in the home in addition to the air filter and vacuum cleaner discussed previously. These steps include reducing mold growth by lowering humidity levels to 25 percent to 50 percent with a dehumidifier. Remember that the dehumidifier must be cleaned and emptied regularly.

Mold growth is highest in warmer months, so an air conditioner can be extremely helpful. Attention must be paid to prevent-

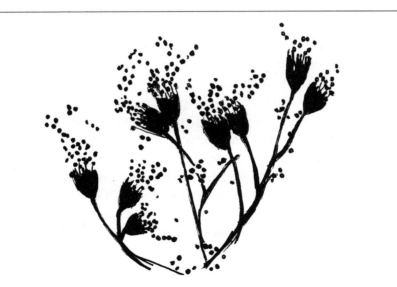

Figure 6.2 Penicillium mold

ing contamination of the air conditioner itself, since any moist area may promote mold growth. Remember the automobile air conditioner, too. Many patients describe allergy and asthma symptoms each time they use their cars' air conditioners due to the exposure to mold. Ventilation is important to reduce mold spore inhalation. An exhaust fan in the bathroom and kitchen to reduce humidity levels is also helpful. Chemical sprays are available to kill mold and prevent its regrowth in areas that are highly susceptible (showers, basements, air conditioners, and so on). The Appendix contains useful information on obtaining these materials. An asthmatic patient should avoid any chemical spray that produces a strong odor, however, and this type of spraying is best done by someone else. Everyone using chemical sprays should use a face mask and make sure there is plenty of ventilation.

Houseplants are not a major source of mold spores but are best kept to a minimum since they increase humidity levels. Spores may also be liberated when the plants are potted or watered.

Animal Allergens

Animal allergens are potent triggers of allergic and asthmatic attacks in sensitive individuals and are commonly found in homes with pets. Exposure to animal allergen such as cat dander may also produce prolonged inflammation of bronchial airways without triggering an attack. If left untreated, this inflammation may lead to severe asthma attacks later.

About 10 percent of the U.S. population is allergic to animals. For persons with asthma the rate is as high as 25 percent. A large proportion of animals surrendered to shelters are from allergic pet owners. Animal allergens may be present in homes or offices even where animals are not kept since allergens can stick to clothing and be carried to any location by the pet's owner. The allergens consist of dander (skin scales) and saliva and are not related to breed or coat length. All breeds of cats, for example, share a common allergen, which may be airborne or present in mattresses, carpets, bed covers, and pillows. An animal's fur, however, may collect allergens such as pollen, dust, and mold and spread these allergens throughout your home. Restricting a pet to a certain room or a portion of the home does not prevent airborne particles from spreading.

Washing your cat or dog weekly will reduce dander levels. This will be difficult at first with cats, but they can be gradually introduced to bathing by starting with one area at a time. An animal's coat can be treated with a spray or solution that reduces exposure to allergens (see the Appendix). With cats remember to wash the face well. Wash your hands after handling your cat and avoid touching your face or eyes. Ensure that your animal is neutered. Wash your clothes and bed linen using detergent solutions at 25°C (77°F) to extract cat allergen.

Even if the pet has been removed from the home, allergens may remain for several months. Cleaning with 3 percent tannic acid solution can denature residual animal allergen. Cat allergen has been demonstrated to remain for years at significant levels in mattresses. Do not forget small pets such as birds and rodents that may produce severe asthmatic attacks in sensitive individuals. A mattress and pillow cover will be helpful in encasing animal allergens. As in the control of dust mites and mold spores, an air filter can be extremely helpful.

Are There Hypoallergenic Pets? A large number of allergic people would like to have a pet for their home but may risk a severe allergic or asthmatic attack. Many are searching for a hypoallergenic pet. One biotechnology company hopes to genetically engineer a hypoallergenic cat in the next several years. Until then individuals can look for animals that are less likely to produce allergic reactions but must accept the fact that all animals produce allergens.

Dogs. Some dog allergens are breed-specific, and some breeds produce less allergen than others. Poodles, Airedales, and schnauzers, for example, produce less allergen since they shed their skin about every twenty-one days. Breeds such as cocker spaniels, German shepherds, and Irish setters shed their skin every three to four days and produce more allergen. The American Kennel Club has listed dog breeds that they consider to be most suitable for allergic people. These include the poodle, labradoodle, bichon frise, Havanese (see Figure 6.3), miniature schnauzer, kerry blue terrier,

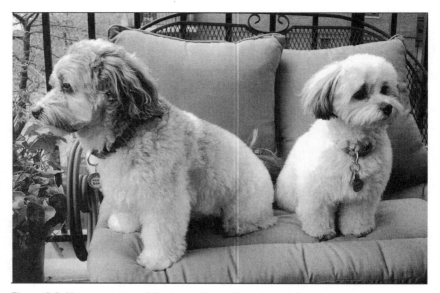

Figure 6.3 Havanese, one of the hypoallergenic breeds of dog

wheaten terrier, Maltese, Portuguese water dog, Italian greyhound, Basenji, Chinese crested, Chihuahua, and Mexican hairless.

Cats. Male cats produce more allergen than females, and neutered males produce less than non-neutered males (with some exceptions). Kittens produce less allergen than adult cats, which may explain why allergic symptoms may not occur until there have been several days or weeks of continuous exposure to the kitten. A study of 321 patients with allergies showed that dark-colored cats were four times more likely to cause more allergic reactions than light-colored cats. Many allergic people report more or less allergic reactions to individual cats.

Before Getting a Pet. It is advisable to have allergy testing (radio-allergosorbent test [RAST] or skin testing) for cat or dog allergen before obtaining your pet. If you are highly allergic then it is inadvisable to proceed. Research the breed you are interested in. Some breeders may allow you to spend time with your prospective pet before you purchase the animal, and many have a return policy.

Cockroaches

Allergy to cockroaches is thought to stem from exposure to the feces, saliva, and bodies of these insects. These substances are commonly found in house dust, particularly in urban locations. A recent study of asthma occurring in a large city found a strong connection between allergy to cockroaches and the number of asthmatic attacks. The increased frequency of asthma as well as fatal asthmatic attacks in the United States has been predominantly in inner-city residents. As many as 60 percent of urban asthmatics are allergic to cockroaches. All asthmatics should be aware of this potential allergy and if cockroaches are present in their homes, invoke control measures. These measures should include control of sources of food and water, routine cleaning, and regular use of insecticides such as hydramethylnon and avermectin in the form of bait.

Reducing Indoor Pollution

Asthma attacks may be precipitated indoors by airborne irritants that are not allergens. In the home, commonly found irritants include tobacco smoke, strong odors, and pollutants from gas stoves, wood stoves, and fireplaces.

Active Smoking

Patients with asthma who smoke do not have to look far to find a reason to stop. Cigarette smoking is the leading cause of respiratory illness and death in the United States. All of these illnesses and deaths are preventable. Cigarette smoking may cause permanent damage in the lung, leading to emphysema and chronic bronchitis. It should be clear to the individual with asthma who smokes that this habit may change a reversible disease (asthma) to an irreversible and often fatal disease (emphysema). In addition, cigarette smoking has been shown to increase "irritability" of the bronchial tubes and, therefore, may be considered a cause of asthma. It has been documented that smoking affects the immune system and the defense of the lung against infection. As a result, smokers have higher rates of sinus and bronchial infection than do nonsmokers, and these infections may trigger asthmatic attacks.

Despite these facts and many others that link cigarette smoking to cancer of the lung and other organs, many patients with asthma continue to smoke. Some stop during attacks and resume when they feel better.

How to Stop Smoking. There is no foolproof method to stop smoking, but some measures have proved helpful. A patient should work closely with a physician, reviewing pulmonary function tests that may already show permanent changes, supporting the decision to quit. It also helps to review the benefits of stopping. Studies have documented that patients who stop smoking have a marked reduction in cough, wheezing, expectoration, and shortness of breath. This may occur as soon as one month after stopping. Reports also show that there are fewer infections after smoking cessation and overall improvement in pulmonary function tests. As a first step to stopping, it is often helpful to demonstrate with a peak flow meter that smoking one cigarette can produce a drop in air movement. The next step is to set a "stop date." It can also help to sign a stop-smoking contract with the physician.

A great deal of information has documented the powerful addictive properties of nicotine. Your physician can help you assess your own degree of physical addiction and the role of psychological dependence. For patients with physical addiction, replacement therapy with nicotine in the form of a lozenge, chewing gum, or a patch may be helpful. A low dose of an antidepressant medication, bupropion (Zyban), has also been found to be helpful in smoking cessation. Varenicline (Chantix), a nicotine blocker, has recently been approved by the FDA for smoking cessation. Other measures can be recommended if these are not successful. A psychological dependence can also be treated successfully. In every patient the message must be clear: "You must stop smoking."

Environmental Tobacco Smoke

Nonsmokers are exposed to many of the same injurious agents inhaled by active smokers. The dangers of secondhand tobacco smoke have been widely publicized. Among these dangers is that children exposed to parental secondhand smoke have been found to have more respiratory illnesses, including asthma. Asthmatic children of smokers have been shown to have more frequent attacks. The Environmental Protection Agency (EPA) has reported a higher frequency of asthmatic attacks in up to one million children of cigarette smokers. In the same report the EPA attributed up to three hundred thousand cases of bronchitis and other respiratory infections in small children to their exposure to secondhand smoke. Environmental tobacco smoke is one of the most frequent triggers of asthmatic attacks reported by patients. In sensitive individuals, even brief inhalation of secondhand smoke may precipitate a severe asthmatic attack.

Asthmatic individuals frequently report that household family members continue to smoke despite the patient's illness. Often the smoking individual will report that they only smoke "in another room." Separating smokers and nonsmokers in the home or workplace does not eliminate exposure to secondhand smoke. To reduce exposure, smoking must be completely prohibited or restricted to a separately ventilated area in order to provide protection for all nonsmokers and especially those with bronchial asthma.

Wood Smoke

Wood smoke from wood-burning stoves and fireplaces also may be an irritant and aggravate bronchial asthma. Approximately 6 percent of homes in the United States have wood stoves and 19 percent have fireplaces. Although the smoke from wood stoves and fireplaces is vented to the outdoors, emissions are found to contaminate indoor air during start-up and when stoking. Particulate matter may also be produced from these sources, which may irritate bronchial asthma. Good ventilation is essential, and an air filter will be helpful if a stove cannot be removed.

Gas Stoves

Gas stoves also may be a source of indoor pollution. Several airborne irritants may be released by gas combustion, including nitrogen dioxide. Although some studies have not found an association between gas stoves and asthma, a recent report suggests that gas stoves may aggravate asthma. As a rule, asthmatic patients should avoid gas and wood-burning stoves.

Formaldehyde and Other Indoor Pollutants

Formaldehyde and other compounds that exist as vapors are found indoors as emissions from construction materials, furnishings such as carpeting, and insulation. Formaldehyde is used in many products including cosmetics, toiletries, medications, and preservatives in some foods. This compound is known to be irritating to the lining of the nose and bronchial tubes, and cases of occupational asthma due to formaldehyde have been reported. At this time, it is not clear how great a role formaldehyde and similar compounds play in aggravating bronchial asthma. To minimize your risk of exposure to these vapors, building materials and furnishings can be selected that do not contain formaldehyde and that have low rates of emission of similar compounds. Ventilation can be increased in areas that are suspected or known to have increased amounts of these substances. Existing sources of formaldehyde such as carpeting can be removed from the home or office. Cleaning solutions, gasoline, and similar materials are best stored in a separate area with excellent ventilation.

Asthmatic attacks have been demonstrated to occur frequently when patients are exposed to strong odors. Simple cooking odors may be extremely irritating. Household sprays, especially those used for cleaning, are often sources of irritation. Other examples include insecticide sprays, deodorants, hair sprays, and perfumes. Paint fumes can be extremely irritating and should be avoided. The simple measures of ensuring adequate ventilation and using an air filter will provide relief from many of these odors if they cannot be avoided.

Ozone and Other Air Pollutants

Air pollutants such as ozone and sulfur dioxide may be found in the home. The levels of these gases are lower indoors than outdoors but still may be irritating to patients with asthma and other lung diseases. As discussed previously, ionizing air filters have been shown to produce ozone. Fine particle pollutants may also be found in the home. Patients should be aware of pollution levels and air pollution "alerts" issued by local public health authorities. Air conditioning can be effective in reducing irritating airborne gases. An air filter reduces levels of particulate pollutants.

Outdoor Allergens and Irritants

Avoidance is the best way to reduce your number of asthmatic attacks triggered by exposure to pollens, molds, and other outdoor allergens. Sensitive individuals are best protected in an air-conditioned environment that contains an air filter. Pollen and mold spore counts are commonly found in newspapers and on TV weather reports so patients can be prepared.

Pollens and Molds

Pollens are seasonal and patients should be able to prepare ahead for particularly difficult months. Patients with known tree pollen allergy who are symptomatic in the spring, for example, may reduce the frequency of asthma attacks by beginning an anti-inflammatory agent such as inhaled corticosteroid or cromolyn or nedocromil two to three weeks before the start of their "season." Those who are sensitive to grasses and ragweed will want to maintain their medication through to the first frost.

Mold spores are more plentiful in warmer months. Thousands of different species of mold exist. They may be found in high numbers on both dry and rainy days. Alternaria is a mold often found in dry, warm climates and in farming areas. Fusarium mold is often found in plants and is abundant during damp, humid weather. Other molds are found in decaying wood and soil. Be sure you anticipate exposure during outdoor activities (mowing the lawn, raking leaves, etc.). A simple filter mask may help you reduce your exposure. Patients may also reduce exposure by staying indoors and using air conditioning and air filtration.

Air Pollution

Air pollution has been demonstrated to have significant adverse effects on patients with lung disease and especially those with bronchial asthma. The EPA has set standards for most common pollutants, including sulfur dioxide (SO_2), nitrogen dioxide (NO_2), carbon monoxide, ozone, particulates, and lead. Sulfur dioxide and particulates are produced by combustion of sulfur-containing fuels such as coal and petroleum. Sulfur dioxide is found in high concentrations near steel mills, power plants, and other factories that burn coal or oil. Particulates are the soot and ashes produced by incinerators, smokestacks, and diesel trucks.

Nitrogen dioxide is a product of industry found in high concentrations when fuel is burned, and it may be released by power plants and automobiles. This type of industrial pollution affects primarily the central and eastern United States but also may be found in any area with many vehicles. According to the EPA, heavy-duty diesel engines produce 25 percent of all vehicle-generated nitrogen oxides, a main component of acid rain and a major source of urban smog. Carbon monoxide is also emitted by automobiles and factories.

Asthmatics are extremely sensitive to sulfur dioxide and may react to exposure with constriction of the bronchial tubes to increased levels of this gas in outdoor air. Increased levels of particulate pollution also have been associated with exacerbations of chronic respiratory disease. The effect of particulate pollution depends on the size and chemical nature of the inhaled particles. Smaller particles have a greater likelihood of reaching the lungs of patients with asthma, bronchitis, and emphysema. A recent study links particulate pollution with a greater likelihood of death from respiratory disease.

Photochemical pollution, or "smog," is the product of the action of sunlight on vehicle exhaust and chemical fumes. Ozone is a product of this interaction and can be used as an index for this type of pollution. Southern California was the first area affected by photochemical pollution, but it has become common in major cities throughout the United States, especially in the summer. Ozone has been shown to cause a reduction in lung function in normal subjects and individuals with asthma. It has been suggested that prolonged exposure may produce chronic lung disease.

National standards for air pollutants have been set with a "margin of safety" that should protect the health of patients with asthma and other illnesses as well as the general population. Air pollution "alerts" are issued by local public health agencies when increased levels of pollution are noted. Air pollutants will be found in greater amounts when weather conditions produce stagnant air circulation. The warm summer months in the eastern United States are particularly dangerous due to increased ozone levels. Patients are advised to stay indoors in an air-conditioned environment during periods of increased pollution. Outdoor exercise, which increases the likelihood of inhaling pollutants, especially should be avoided during these periods. Remember that pollutants such as ozone may also be damaging to individuals with healthy lungs and, therefore, should be avoided by everyone.

Air Temperature

Patients should also consider air temperature. Cold air is extremely irritating to patients with bronchial asthma and may produce severe attacks. When breathing, individuals with asthma appear to warm cold air less quickly and efficiently. This warming normally takes place in the large air passages of the nose, sinuses, throat, and windpipe. One simple measure patients should take is to wrap the face with a scarf that warms air before it is inhaled. A cold air mask is commercially available (see the Appendix) and may provide more protection in the winter.

How to Avoid Severe or Fatal Asthma Attacks

Patients who experience severe or near-fatal asthma attacks must be active participants in monitoring and managing their asthma. Several characteristics of fatal or near-fatal asthma attacks stand out and are emphasized here.

There is usually a period of falling airflows and increased wheezing, cough, and shortness of breath that precedes a severe attack. In this critical time the introduction of oral corticosteroid or an adjustment of maintenance treatment may prevent a near-fatal asthma attack. Unfortunately, patients with severe and subsequently fatal asthma often experience denial of their condition and symptoms. These patients are particularly vulnerable to fatal attacks, since they often disregard instructions to monitor flows and take medications. Usually, these patients admit to self-medication without communication with the physician, lowering dosages or omitting entirely oral and inhaled corticosteroids (for fear of side effects despite a life-threatening disease), and reducing the number of sprays from the recommended dosages of β-agonists, cromolyn, and nedocromil.

It is not clear why these patients place themselves at greater risk through denial of their disease and lack of communication with physicians. Unfortunate childhood experiences may play a role in how an adult deals with disease. Poor rapport with the physician or lack of detailed understanding of the nature of asthma may also be factors. It is only through education that patients may reach a better understanding of the potential severity and life-threatening aspects of bronchial asthma. Professional counseling may be necessary to reduce denial and to enlighten patients as to why they often do not follow instructions.

It has been reported that patients who have had near-fatal asthma attacks may have a reduced perception of shortness of breath. These patients may also have less response to reduced blood oxygen levels. These characteristics would make fatal attacks more likely. By carefully monitoring peak flows, these patients stand a better chance of recognizing the increased narrowing of airways that signals an asthma attack. When flows are reduced 25 percent from the patient's personal best, action must be taken at once. Written instructions help ensure an appropriate response.

Who Is Most Likely to Experience a Fatal Attack?

Patients who have already experienced a severe attack that required respiratory support are the likeliest candidates for fatal asthmatic attacks. When respiratory support is needed, the patient's airway or windpipe is intubated with a tube connected to a mechanical ventilator or respirator. Another characteristic that identifies "high-risk" patients is an extremely variable or unstable airflow. These patients may have peak flows that drop or increase precipitously. Patients who have required frequent courses of oral corticosteroids or who are maintained on oral steroids should also be considered at greater risk for severe attacks.

About 10 percent to 25 percent of all deaths from asthma occur within three hours after the onset of an attack. These patients may progress from minimal symptoms to a collapse of their respirations in a short time. Investigators term this malady "sudden asphyxic asthma." For most patients there is a longer period during which the patient and physician can detect deterioration and instability and act quickly to avoid severe and near-fatal episodes. Without careful home monitoring of peak flows and close communication and compliance with physician instructions, patients who are at high risk for severe asthmatic attacks are likely to experience repeated episodes.

A Case of Fatal Asthma

Several years ago I received a message to call a New York City policeman about the discovery of the body of a sixty-six-year-old woman who had been under my care for asthma. The patrolman had been called by neighbors to enter the patient's apartment since she was not answering her door or phone. A number of people had seen her enter her building in some distress. She had used her bronchodilator spray in the lobby of her building and had not been seen or heard from since. When the policeman and neighbors entered the apartment they found my patient in a chair, still in her overcoat, clutching her bronchodilator spray. The patient had apparently died soon after entering her apartment.

This patient was a delightful woman who edited a foreign policy journal. Office visits were often forums for discussion of a number of topics, and she enjoyed debating different points of view. Unfortunately, she had severe asthma that required frequent courses of corticosteroid as well as a long list of other medications. I had seen her about a month before she died, noted significant wheezing, and prescribed oral corticosteroids. She was afraid of further steroid use and resisted. "I can just use my asthma spray a little more and I'll be all right." Further discussion revealed she had stopped or reduced a number of her medicines on her own ("I don't think I need them").

Fatal asthma is always tragic since it usually can be prevented. I often wonder what the outcome would have been if this patient had taken her prescribed medication. A number of physicians have said, "No one should die of asthma." Unfortunately, these deaths still occur.

Support Systems

In managing bronchial asthma, it helps the patient to have a support system. This is particularly beneficial for patients with moderate or severe asthma who may need emergency care.

Adult Patients

For adults the support system should include a "care partner" who is aware of the patient's illness, physician's name and phone number, and pharmacy number and who has access to a list of the patient's medications as well as the written instructions that the patient has received from the physician. The patient as well as the care partner should know the location of the nearest emergency room in case of a severe attack. Patients should choose carefully their care partners in terms of proximity and accessibility.

A support group may also be helpful for adult patients with bronchial asthma. Patients with asthma may have experienced severe attacks and have fears concerning future episodes and dependency on medication. In addition, patients may fear exercising and undertaking social activities. Many patients may have been misinformed as to the nature of their illness ("it's all in your head") and have been objects of ridicule. Patients should look to their local lung association or medical society if their physicians are not familiar with a specific program. These support groups should be managed by a physician who is a specialist in respiratory diseases. As noted, the primary source of information should be the patient's physician, but a support group may further the patient's knowledge and ability to cope with this disease. Patients who have difficult problems in these areas may benefit from professional counseling. The primary physician should be the source of a referral.

Children with Asthma

In children with bronchial asthma, parents usually serve as the care partner. It is extremely important that all members of the child's family be aware of the nature of this disease as well as of the treatment needed. Conflicts can be avoided through proper education directed by the child's physician. This education should also be directed to teachers and friends who are involved in the child's daily activities.

Children may have problems accepting that they have an illness that may cause restrictions on their activities. They may suffer embarrassment at school or when playing if attacks occur. The physician and parent must reinforce a positive attitude in the child regarding asthma to avoid loss of self-esteem and development of poor self-image. Emphasis should be placed on maintaining as close to normal as possible activities at home and school, including exercise. This should be understood by teachers as well as parents. The school nurse or physician should be made aware of the child's illness and should have on record the child's physician's name and a list of the child's medications.

Asthma Camps

Support groups for children and parents are available that take the form of "asthma camps" or year-round activities. The physician should be able to direct or advise parents in contacting these groups. See the Appendix for a list of national organizations that can provide names of these groups.

Stress and Asthma

Asthma has often been associated with anxiety and stress to such an extent that many individuals have erroneously attributed the disease to a psychological disorder. A recent study has documented that anxiety occurs no more frequently in patients with bronchial asthma than in the general population. The same appears true for depression.

Anxiety and Depression

In the more severe asthmatic the level of anxiety increases. This is usually due to feelings of breathlessness and chest tightness experienced more frequently by patients with moderate to severe asthma. Patients who have suffered severe attacks and may have had emergency care or hospitalization may also suffer increased anxiety. In addition, depression may develop in a setting of chronic bronchial asthma as with any other chronic illness.

Although anxiety and depression may occur in patients with bronchial asthma, there is no evidence that they cause the disease. It is likely, however, that they are aggravating factors in the course of this illness. Therefore, every effort should be made to reduce stress and to treat anxiety and depression. This is accomplished best by psychological counseling. Relaxation techniques and biofeedback also have been helpful in reducing stress in patients with bronchial asthma. As a rule, tranquilizers should be avoided, since they may affect respiratory drive and decrease awareness of shortness of breath. In addition, some antidepressants may have adverse effects on the respiratory system. Before any medication is prescribed for anxiety and/or depression, there must be close consultation between the primary physician and the consulting psychiatrist.

The Asthma Diet

Patients with bronchial asthma can also participate in their care and management by carefully monitoring their diets. Although there is no extensive evidence that ingestion of a certain food product is beneficial in treatment of asthma, there is evidence that sensitive asthmatics should avoid certain foods, preservatives, and dyes.

Patients who have experienced allergic reactions to specific foods must carefully avoid these products. Immediate reactions may include development of hives (urticaria), wheezing, collapse of the circulation, and swelling of the throat (anaphylaxis). Common sources of allergic or asthmatic reactions include shrimp and other shellfish, eggs, milk, soy, wheat, and peanuts. Asthma attacks triggered by food allergies are much more common in children, particularly those with the allergic skin rash known as eczema. In adults these reactions are much less frequent and do not often trigger asthmatic attacks.

It is important to distinguish between a history of a specific allergic reaction that a patient has experienced and a positive allergy test alone. In many instances a positive allergy test (skin or blood) for a particular food may result despite the fact that the patient has ingested the food without reaction. In patients who have severe, unstable asthma it may be helpful to withdraw this food or food group and observe the patient's response. This should not be necessary in patients with less severe asthma that is well controlled.

Research has suggested that a diet rich in magnesium may be beneficial to lung function and may actually reduce wheezing and bronchial irritability. Magnesium is found in cereals, nuts, green vegetables, and dairy products. In patients who are not sensitive to these products, a diet rich in magnesium may help.

Sulfites

Sulfites are a common food and beverage preservative that may cause asthmatic attacks in sensitive individuals. These preservatives have been used to make products appear "fresh" and reduce spoilage. Salad bars in restaurants were common sources of sulfite exposure until 1986, when the Food and Drug Administration (FDA) banned the use of sulfites on fruits and vegetables served as "fresh." It is believed that the irritant producing the asthmatic reaction is sulfur dioxide gas liberated from salts of sulfite, bisulfite or metabisulfite.

Not all asthmatics are sensitive to sulfites. Sulfite sensitivity may develop at any point in life and is most common in severe asthmatics. As a rule, however, it is best for all asthmatics to avoid sulfites, especially if they have had asthmatic reactions while dining in restaurants ("restaurant asthma"). Patients who are sensitive will have immediate asthmatic reactions. Sulfite reactions may also include stomach pains, hives, and anaphylactic shock. Some of the products containing sulfites that may cause reactions include processed potatoes, baked products, fresh shrimp, fruit drinks, dried fruits, beer, and wine.

Patients with sulfite sensitivity should read food labels carefully and choose foods that do not contain sulfites. In 1986, the FDA ruled that sulfites used specifically as preservatives must be listed on the label. This ruling includes beer and wine bottled since that time. Sulfites that are used in food processing but do not serve as preservatives in the final food must be listed on the label if present at levels of 10 parts per million or higher. Currently, there are six sulfiting agents allowed in packaged foods. The names by which they are listed on food labels are sulfur dioxide, sodium sulfite, sodium and potassium bisulfite, and sodium and potassium metabisulfite.

Sulfites have been used as preservatives in medications, too, including some asthma medications. Some nebulizer solutions, for instance, may contain sulfites. This would explain why some patients may experience wheezing instead of improvement after a nebulizer treatment. For these sulfite-sensitive patients, nebulizer solutions that do not contain sulfites are available.

Tartrazine

Tartrazine, a yellow dye (FD&C Yellow Dye #5) that has been used in foods (e.g., margarine) and medications has been demonstrated to cause asthmatic attacks in certain sensitive individuals. At this time it appears this is a rare reaction affecting only a few patients. Those who have experienced attacks after ingestion of tartrazine should avoid it and check carefully for the presence of this substance in foods and medications.

Do I Have to Change My Job?

When considering how an occupation impacts bronchial asthma, several factors must be considered. The environment may have a substantial influence on asthma. Working outdoors in cold air may trigger asthmatic attacks. High degrees of air pollution with exposure to ozone, sulfur dioxide, and particulates may affect asthmatic workers with outdoor jobs. Patients with known allergies to pollens and mold spores as well as other allergens may have to work in air-conditioned environments.

Occupational asthma will be discussed in detail in Chapter 8. This condition may be created by a work exposure or develop due to worsening of a preexisting condition in the workplace. It is clear that allergic individuals may be likelier to develop occupational asthma. Asthmatic patients should research their occupations for the incidence of work-related illnesses.

Since asthma may worsen with exercise, it is important for a patient to consider how much exertion is required by a particular occupation. Heavy exertion may have to be avoided to reduce the incidence of asthma attacks. Just as the athlete may benefit from premedication with a β_2-agonist or cromolyn sodium before exercise, the worker may also use this approach if high degrees of exertion are required.

With these precautions and adjustments, it should be possible to avoid changing a patient's occupation due to the presence of bronchial asthma.

Do I Have to Move?

In 2006 the Asthma and Allergy Foundation of America ranked the top 100 metropolitan areas in the country based on twelve asthma risk factors, including asthma-related deaths, annual pollen level, annual air quality, public smoking laws, and the number of asthma specialists. Based on these and other factors Scranton, Pennsylvania, topped the list as the worst U.S. asthma city. Richmond, Virginia, and Philadelphia took the second and third spots, and Atlanta was ranked fourth. The best asthma city was Tampa, Florida. See the Appendix for information on the Asthma and Allergy Foundation of America.

People with severe asthma should consider relocation if they find that they are living in one of the worst asthma cities. Mild asthmatics that are under good control should not have to consider moving.

Achieving Your Asthma Goals

One of the treatment goals of bronchial asthma is achieving as normal a lifestyle as possible. Patients who actively participate in their care will often achieve this goal. As noted, participation includes self-monitoring and education, avoidance and elimination of irritating substances from your environment, adjustment of activity and diet, and communication with the physician. These steps require time and effort, but the benefits will certainly be worth it.

7

Asthma and Pregnancy

ASTHMA COMPLICATES 4 percent to 8 percent of all pregnancies and is considered one of the most common serious medical problems that may occur during pregnancy. It is absolutely essential that the control of asthma be maintained throughout pregnancy to protect the health of the mother and her child.

Rationale for Treatment

Treating asthma during pregnancy varies little from the general treatment of bronchial asthma. The basis of this principle is that the developing fetus depends on the maternal circulation for its supply of oxygen. If the mother suffers uncontrolled asthma, oxygen levels are reduced, creating a threat to the unborn child. Therefore, the medications for treating asthma are usually maintained during pregnancy. Any medication judged unnecessary or which is unsafe during pregnancy should be withdrawn.

Complications of Unstable Asthma and Pregnancy

Studies have shown that pregnant women with uncontrolled, unstable asthma have a greater risk for complicated pregnancies. These complications include premature birth, preeclampsia, increased perinatal mortality, and low birth weight. Pregnant women with severe asthma may suffer from high blood pressure, vaginal hemorrhage, and toxemia. They also may have induced or complicated labor. Women with well-controlled asthma have decreased risk of developing these complications.

Diagnosing Asthma During Pregnancy

Asthma may occur for the first time during pregnancy. The diagnosis may be obscured because shortness of breath is common in pregnancy. Increased progesterone levels in pregnancy seem to stimulate respiration, resulting in hyperventilation and shortness of breath. This may occur early in pregnancy. In the later stages of pregnancy, shortness of breath is also common due to enlargement of the uterus limiting full inspiration. Asthma may still be diagnosed correctly, however, with a thorough history and physical exam combined with spirometry. Flow rate measurements remain accurate in pregnancy even in the third trimester when lung volumes may be reduced by enlargement of the uterus. Oxygen measurements are particularly useful in monitoring asthma during pregnancy. This may be done easily with the pulse oximeter. Any significant decrease in oxygen levels must be closely followed and reversed through aggressive treatment.

Monitoring Asthma During Pregnancy

The course of asthma has been found to change in about two-thirds of women during pregnancy. Therefore, monthly evaluations of asthma symptoms and lung function are recommended. Spirometry is preferred on follow-up visits but measurement of peak flows (see Chapter 3) may suffice.

Fetal Monitoring. Once pregnancy is confirmed, a patient's obstetrician and the physician responsible for the treatment of the patient's asthma should confer. In view of the potential for complications during pregnancy, fetal monitoring will be stressed. In women with moderate or severe asthma this monitoring will include early ultrasonography (at twelve to twenty weeks). In these patients and those who have had frequent asthma attacks during pregnancy, this procedure and monitoring of the fetal heart rate will be repeated frequently during the third trimester. Ultrasound examination may also be helpful after a severe asthma exacerbation.

Course of Asthma During Pregnancy

The course of asthma during pregnancy has been the subject of study. Just as the disease varies from patient to patient, the severity of asthma during pregnancy will also vary. Approximately a third of patients will suffer worsening of their symptoms while the rest will improve or stay the same. This course also appears to be consistent for subsequent pregnancies. If asthma worsens it often happens between twenty-four and thirty-six weeks of the pregnancy with subsequent improvement. Exacerbations during labor and delivery are rare. Approximately three months postpartum, patients will usually return to the degree of asthma they were experiencing prior to pregnancy.

Treating Asthma During Pregnancy

The general principles of maintaining good control of bronchial asthma should be vigorously applied throughout pregnancy. Patients should maintain their environmental control precautions and avoid as many allergens as possible. (See Chapter 6.) Peak flows should be recorded daily, and medications maintained and adjusted accordingly. Understandably, there is a natural reluctance to take medications during pregnancy, but, in general, asthma medications have been found to be safe during pregnancy and should be continued under the guidance of the physician in consultation with the patient's obstetrician.

General Guidelines: Preferred Medications

The data on the effects of the asthma drugs during pregnancy come from both human and animal studies. The results of animal studies should be reviewed with the knowledge that effects noted in animals may not apply to humans. Some general guidelines for use of asthma drugs can be applied. Inhaled medications are preferred since these agents do not have as much total body effect as oral or injectable agents. As a rule, medications that have been in use longer are also preferred since there is greater experience with their use. Preferred medications for pregnant women are listed in Table 7.1. For a more extensive discussion of these medications, refer to Chapter 4.

B$_2$-Agonists. The inhaled β$_2$-agonists are the first-line bronchodilators for as-needed use during pregnancy. As a group, there is extensive human experience with no evidence of fetal injury. Animal studies are also generally without evidence for adverse effects except at high doses. The greatest experience has been with albuterol (Proventil, Ventolin), which is the preferred agent. There is too little data on the use of levalbuterol (Xopenex) in pregnancy to recommend its use. When given by inhalation in normal dosages, β$_2$-agonists may be used safely throughout pregnancy, labor, and delivery. The β$_2$-agonists may also be used orally and by nebulization if deemed necessary. In patients with mild asthma (no more than two attacks a week and no nocturnal attacks), the β$_2$-agonists may be adequate for controlling the patient's bronchial asthma during pregnancy.

The long-acting β$_2$-agonists, salmeterol (Serevent) and formoterol (Foradil), have limited data on their use in pregnancy. Their similarity to short-acting agents suggests that they may be used during pregnancy but only if indicated by the severity of the mother's asthma.

Avoid Nonselective Agents. Nonselective β-agonists are best avoided during pregnancy. These agents, such as epinephrine (adrenaline) and isoproterenol, have both beta-1 and beta-2 effects. Animal studies of these agents have demonstrated abnormal embryo development. Reports from human studies have raised questions concerning their safety. In view of the fact that the selective β$_2$-agonists are available, there is no need to use nonselective medications.

Theophylline. Theophylline may also be used as a bronchodilator in pregnancy. There is extensive favorable human experience with this agent. Theophylline may be used intravenously as aminophylline in an emergency. It is essential that blood levels be monitored closely during pregnancy, and it is recommended that theophylline levels not be greater than 12 mg/L, since infants born of women with higher levels have been found to have adverse effects of theophylline, such as jitteriness, vomiting, and rapid heartbeat.

Anticholinergic Agents. The anticholinergic agents ipratropium bromide (Atrovent) and tiotropium bromide (Spiriva) have not been studied in humans during pregnancy. Animal studies of ipratropium bromide, however, have not shown any evidence of abnormal fetal development. Since these agents are also relatively weak bronchodilators in asthmatic patients, they are not preferred for use during pregnancy.

Table 7.1   Preferred Asthma Drugs During Pregnancy

Bronchodilator

Short-acting inhaled β_2-agonist: Albuterol

If oral β_2-agonist needed: Terbutaline

Long-acting β_2-agonist for moderate to severe asthma

Theophylline if needed (keep level 8–12 mg/L)

Anti-Inflammatory Agent

Inhaled corticosteroid: Budesonide*

Alternatives: Cromolyn

Oral corticosteroid: Prednisone for severe exacerbation

For Associated Conditions

Allergic rhinitis: Budesonide, cromolyn, loratadine, or cetirizine

Bacterial infection (such as sinusitis): Amoxicillin (use erythromycin if allergic to penicillin)

*Patients under good control on other inhaled corticosteroids may continue these agents.

Inhaled Corticosteroids. Anti-inflammatory agents are also needed during pregnancy for patients with more than mild, intermittent asthma. Inhaled corticosteroids are the preferred anti-inflammatory agent that can be used safely during pregnancy. Of the agents available in the United States, the greatest human experience has been with budesonide (Pulmicort). Large studies of inhaled corticosteroids during pregnancy have shown no increase in congenital malformations or other adverse perinatal outcomes. These same studies have demonstrated that inhaled corticosteroids reduce the risk of asthma exacerbations during pregnancy and improve lung function.

Systemic Corticosteroids. Systemic corticosteroids (oral and injectable) may also be needed to treat severe asthma attacks during pregnancy. These agents may be used safely and should not be withheld due to fear of adverse effects on a patient's pregnancy. Human studies have shown only a slight increase in preeclampsia, low birth weight, and premature births in patients receiving systemic corticosteroids for prolonged periods throughout pregnancy. In large human studies, there has been no clear evidence of increased birth defects secondary to the use of corticosteroids during pregnancy.

Cromolyn Sodium. Cromolyn sodium (Intal) is a nonsteroidal anti-inflammatory agent that may be used safely during pregnancy. Both human and animal studies have had favorable results. Cromolyn should be regarded as an alternative anti-inflammatory agent to inhaled corticosteroids during pregnancy.

Nedocromil Sodium. Nedocromil sodium (Tilade) resembles cromolyn and is another nonsteroidal anti-inflammatory agent. Although animal studies are favorable, at this time there is no human experience to refer to. For this reason, cromolyn sodium would be the preferred alternative to inhaled corticosteroids.

Anti-Leukotrienes. Anti-leukotrienes have not been used extensively in pregnant women. Although data from animal testing have been reassuring, these agents would not be preferred during pregnancy.

Step Therapy for Asthma During Pregnancy

Mild Intermittent Asthma. Short-acting β_2-agonists are recommended on an as-needed basis in people with intermittent asthma. Albuterol is the preferred agent due to its excellent safety profile and the large amount of data on its use during pregnancy.

Mild Persistent Asthma. The regular use of low-dose inhaled corticosteroids is recommended for people with mild persistent asthma. Budesonide is the preferred agent, but there is no evidence that the other inhaled corticosteroids are unsafe during pregnancy. Patients who are under good control with these agents may continue them.

Cromolyn, anti-leukotrienes, and theophylline are alternatives to inhaled corticosteroids but are not preferred.

Moderate Persistent Asthma. There are two preferred treatment options for people with moderate persistent asthma: (1) a combination of low-dose inhaled corticosteroid and a long-acting β_2-agonist or (2) an increase to medium-dose inhaled corticosteroids. There is only a small amount of data comparing these two options in pregnancy but when the comparison has been made in nonpregnant adults, the combination option has been more effective.

Severe Persistent Asthma. Individuals with severe persistent asthma require a high dose of inhaled corticosteroid in combination with a long-acting β_2-agonist. If asthma symptoms persist, oral corticosteroids should be added.

Should Allergy Treatments Be Started or Continued?

Immunotherapy (also called desensitization) has been helpful in reducing asthma attacks in allergic patients, although adverse reactions to allergy injections may occur in sensitive individuals. A severe, total body reaction such as anaphylaxis would threaten a developing fetus. Anaphylaxis has also been reported to induce labor. For these reasons it is recommended that no allergy treatment or immunotherapy be started during pregnancy.

In patients who have reached maintenance therapy in which dosages of allergens injected are not increased and who are not known to have reactions, immunotherapy may continue as prescribed by the patient's physician. Patients who are extremely sensitive and who have had systemic reactions such as anaphylaxis are best not treated.

Treating Related Conditions During Pregnancy
Allergic Rhinitis and Sinusitis

There is a high incidence of allergic rhinitis and sinusitis in patients with bronchial asthma, and there is a greater frequency of sinusitis during pregnancy. Upper and lower respiratory tract infections, including pneumonia, may occur during pregnancy. Treatment of these conditions should not be delayed since they may trigger more severe asthma attacks. Many medications can be used safely for these conditions, while some should definitely be avoided.

Intranasal Sprays. Allergic rhinitis such as hay fever may be treated with intranasal topical corticosteroid sprays as well as intranasal cromolyn sodium. Of the intranasal steroids, budesonide (Rhinocort Aqua) is the preferred agent due to its large human experience. The aerosol spray treatments are preferred over oral antihistamines.

Antibiotics. Antibiotics may be needed during pregnancy to treat specific infections. Indiscriminate use of antibiotics should be avoided, especially when viral infection is most likely as in the common cold. Tetracycline, sulfonamides (in late pregnancy), and the quinolones should be avoided during pregnancy. Penicillin and its derivatives such as amoxicillin may be used safely. For penicillin-allergic patients, erythromycin may be substituted. Sulfonamides may be used in early or midpregnancy.

Antihistamines. First-generation antihistamines, such as chlorpheniramine and diphenhydramine, may be used safely during pregnancy but may cause drowsiness. The second-generation antihistamines, loratadine (Claritin) and cetirizine (Zyrtec), are preferred during pregnancy.

Decongestants. Decongestants may be indicated to relieve persistent and severe nasal symptoms in rhinitis and the common cold. Human experience with pseudoephredrine has been favorable, although animal studies have shown fetal abnormalities. An alternative is oxymetazoline nasal spray or drops for a period not to exceed five days. One drawback to oxymetazoline is a patient's tendency to become dependent on its decongestant effect from prolonged use.

The Common Cold

Some simple measures can help treat the common cold. A buffered saline nasal spray can moisturize irritated nasal membranes and flush dried mucus. Patients should force fluids; warm fluids provide some relief from nasal congestion. Bed rest can also help and often shortens recovery. For severe nasal symptoms the decongestants may be helpful. All treatment should be directed by the patient's physician. Any persistent fever, sore throat, sinus pain, and discharge should prompt quick examination and treatment. Cultures can be obtained to document bacterial infections that will require antibiotic therapy.

In many instances a common cold triggers increased bronchial narrowing, which may occur through throat and bronchial infections as well as through irritation of the bronchial tubes by postnasal discharge. Peak flows should be monitored closely during colds to identify when bronchoconstriction occurs. Early recognition of bronchial narrowing allows the patient and physician to begin a treatment plan that reverses bronchoconstriction before a severe attack can occur. This plan may include an increase in the number of sprays of a topical corticosteroid or a course of oral steroid.

Is Flu Vaccine Safe During Pregnancy?

A killed vaccine, such as influenza vaccine, does not pose a threat during pregnancy. In fact, it is a good idea for patients with moderate to severe asthma to receive influenza vaccine in order to avoid this severe infection that may exacerbate their disease. This vaccine should be administered before December 1 in order to allow enough time for antibody levels to become effective.

Labor and Delivery

All of the preferred asthma medications can be continued during labor. In general, patients should continue their normal asthma medications throughout labor. Corticosteroids may also be given in those patients who have been steroid dependent and may have adrenal insufficiency. The type of delivery will be determined by the patient's obstetrician. In patients with severe or unstable asthma, a cesarean section may be necessary.

A thirty-four-year-old woman with severe asthma has been under my care for twenty-four years. Sixteen years ago she asked me if I thought it was medically safe for her to have a child. The patient had been hospitalized for asthma and had required frequent courses of oral corticosteroids. Her daily treatment plan included regular β_2-agonist, inhaled corticosteroid, cromolyn sodium, and theophylline. We decided to do a detailed pulmonary function test to help in the decision. I knew that she was highly motivated and involved in her care. She was also extremely compliant with her medication routine and called whenever there was a significant drop in her peak flow. I reviewed her breathing tests and found that her lung capacity was 70 percent of normal after she used her bronchodilator spray. The patient's oxygen level was near normal. I told her that I thought she could become pregnant. During her pregnancy she required oral corticosteroids several times and maintained her usual medications. I spoke frequently with her obstetrician. The patient's asthma remained severe but did not worsen, and she delivered a healthy baby girl by cesarean section. Her asthma has remained severe and during office visits we sometimes refer to her daughter as the "miracle baby." When I look back at all the factors that had to be considered, I am sure I would make the same decision.

After Delivery

Asthma medications are commonly found in breast milk but that should not keep asthmatic mothers from breast-feeding. The inhaled medications (β_2-agonists, inhaled corticosteroids, cromolyn sodium) do not reach significant levels in breast milk and should have little, if any, effect on an infant. Oral corticosteroids are secreted in breast milk, but only a small fraction of the mother's dosage reaches the infant. Prednisone and prednisolone are also considered compatible with breast-feeding. Theophylline is secreted in breast milk but less than 1 percent of the mother's dose ever reaches the child. In rare instances, excessive irritability has been reported in infants being breast-fed by mothers receiving theophylline. If that occurs and the mother's asthma is well controlled, it is usually possible to interrupt theophylline and adjust other medications.

Avoiding Complications During Pregnancy

To reduce complications that may adversely affect the mother and developing child, asthma should be well controlled before and during pregnancy. Uncontrolled asthma may reduce oxygen delivery to the fetus and lead to serious complications. Treatment of asthma during pregnancy is similar to the general treatment plan discussed in Chapter 5. Most of the asthma medications are clearly safe during pregnancy and should be used normally. Certain medications are preferred and they are listed in this chapter. Unfortunately, fear of medication side effects during pregnancy has prompted many asthmatic patients to eliminate their medicines, thus increasing their risk of complications. Through patient education and communication with the physician as well as careful use of asthma medications, the risk of complications for pregnant asthmatics can be greatly reduced.

8

Occupational Asthma

THERE IS LITTLE doubt that asthma may develop or worsen in the workplace, creating a significant health problem. Estimates of the incidence of occupational asthma vary according to the industry. Each year new agents that may cause asthma are identified and another occupation is added to an expanding list. At last count more than 250 agents had been identified as potential causes of occupational asthma. In a forty-hour workweek it is estimated that the air passages from the nose to the air sacs of the lung come into contact with 14,000 liters of air in the workplace. With exertion this amount of air increases twelve times with a greater amount bypassing the nose, which acts as a filter. Strong irritants (such as ammonia) may signal a reaction, but many materials (such as asbestos) pass into the lung without an individual's knowledge and may produce severe injury.

What Is Occupational Asthma?

Occupational asthma is an illness created in the workplace by a particular material. Work-related asthma can be an exacerbation of preexisting disease (work-aggravated asthma) or the new onset of asthma caused by exposure to an increasing number of irritates or sensitizing materials. These offending agents occur in many forms, including animal and vegetable proteins, dyes, chemicals, particulates, propellants, and enzymes. These agents can produce reactions by direct contact or through forms such as dusts, vapors, or powders.

Work-Aggravated Asthma

Work-aggravated asthma is caused by direct irritation of the airways from dust and chemicals. Examples include acidic or alkaline cleaning solutions or powders, rock and mineral dusts, cement dust, ammonia, ozone, and volatile organic compounds found in paints and solvents.

New Onset Asthma in the Workplace

In new onset asthma developed in the workplace, exposure to biologic proteins (particles from wood products, textiles, and grains) stimulate the production of Immunoglobulin E (IgE) specific for these materials. A subsequent exposure triggers the release of chemical mediators that produce the asthmatic reaction. People with known allergy or who smoke are at greater risk of developing this form of occupational asthma. Additional materials may produce new onset asthma in the workplace without the production of a specific IgE. These include isocyanates, which are widely used in polyurethane foams and paints and are frequently recognized as a cause of occupational asthma.

A single heavy exposure of a highly irritating material, such as chlorine gas, bleach, strong acids, and contaminants in metalworking fluids, may produce the sudden onset of asthma in the workplace.

Some Examples of Occupational Asthma

Farmers or veterinarians may develop asthma as a result of sensitization to proteins in animal hair, dander, and urine. Bakers may develop asthma as a result of reactions to flour. Woodworkers may become sensitized to dusts from various woods and develop asthmatic reactions. Butchers who handle plastic wraps may become sensitized to the material. A worker in the plastics and paint industries may be exposed to toluene diisocyanate (TDI), which has been shown to be particularly sensitizing. Beauticians may develop asthma as a reaction to chemicals and sprays used in their work. Even these few examples of occupational asthma demonstrate how significant this problem may be for workers and industry. A more complete list is in Table 8.1.

Latex Allergy: On the Rise

A striking and often severe example of occupational asthma occurs from exposure to latex. Allergy to latex has increased dramatically in the last two decades. This increase is directly related to the AIDS

Table 8.1   *Examples of Occupational Asthma*

Occupation or Industry	Agents
Baker	Flours, cottonseed oil
Beautician	Fluorocarbon propellants, persulfate
Carpenter, wood worker	Wood dust
Farmer	Soybean dust
Grocery worker	Plastic wrapping
Hospital worker	Latex, psyllium, disinfectants
Pesticide worker	Organophosphates
Pharmaceutical worker	Antibiotics, lactose
Plastics, paint worker	Toluene diisocyanate
Postal worker, bookbinder	Glue (fish origin)
Poultry worker	Animal proteins, aprolium
Printer	Vegetable gums
Refinery worker	Platinum salts, vanadium
Textile worker	Cotton, flax, hemp dust
Veterinarian, laboratory worker	Animal dander, urine
Welder	Stainless steel fumes

epidemic of the 1980s, which prompted a tremendous increase in the use of latex gloves. It is estimated that since 1980, the number of people in the general population with latex allergy has increased from 1 percent to 8 percent. Among dental workers, the number with latex sensitivity has increased from 7 percent to 40 percent, while other health care workers have experienced an increase from 3 percent to 20 percent.

In order to produce allergy, latex proteins must enter the body. The most common source is the powdered cornstarch used in latex gloves. The latex protein combines with this powder during manufacturing. Patients breathe in this dust when the gloves are slipped on. Latex protein also may enter the body through direct contact so that allergic reactions may occur during or after surgery or other medical procedures.

Latex-induced asthma is often severe, requiring health care workers to leave their occupations. Many health care centers have taken steps to reduce latex exposure through the use of nonlatex, powderless gloves. Latex gloves, however, are still used in most surgeries since they provide the best protection against infection. Allergy testing for latex is widely available, so anyone who suspects the presence of this allergy in the workplace should be tested.

When Should I Suspect I May Have Occupational Asthma?

A history of onset of asthma after a new workplace exposure or an exacerbation of preexisting asthma indicates that the asthma may be work-related. The basis for such a diagnosis comes from a thorough occupational history linked to physical and laboratory findings under the direction of a physician. But the patient is the one who calls medical symptoms to the attention of the physician. A high degree of awareness helps identify what may be occupational sources of asthma.

Look for "Monday Morning Asthma"

There may be clues that should prompt further investigation into the possibility of occupational asthma. The symptoms of cough, eye irritation, and nasal congestion may occur at work before the wheezing or shortness of breath develops. These symptoms often occur only at work and not in any other environment. The longer a worker is exposed, however, the greater the likelihood of persistent symptoms outside the workplace. "Monday morning asthma" is a term that describes the sudden onset of symptoms when workers return to work. Symptoms may decline somewhat during the week with a great improvement on weekends or during vacations or other absences. Although many reactions are immediate, it is important to recall the late phase of bronchial asthma and how reactions may be delayed and occur hours after leaving the workplace.

Can Occupational Asthma Become Chronic?

Studies have demonstrated that the longer the patient is exposed to the offending agent the more likely the asthma will become chronic. Without information on an individual's occupation (obtained when recording a patient's medical history) it is easy to see how occupational asthma might be overlooked. Even after a worker leaves a job that has produced occupational asthma, the symptoms may continue for years.

Therapy for occupational asthma, therefore, must emphasize prevention, early diagnosis, and removal of the substance responsible for the exposure.

How You Can Help Make the Diagnosis

Patients may be asked by their physicians to aid in the diagnosis of occupational asthma. Valuable information can be obtained by using a peak flow meter. Readings of airflows at home and at work may document precipitous drops in the workplace or hours after exposure. This type of "challenge test" is preferred to a laboratory study in which a physician attempts to duplicate workplace conditions. In establishing the diagnosis of asthma, a bronchial challenge test (see Chapter 2) may also be used to document airway overreactivity, a characteristic of asthma. Laboratory testing may also be helpful with radioallergosorbent testing (RAST) that may target specific substances found in the individual's workplace. It should be remembered that a positive reaction, however, confirms sensitivity but does not demonstrate airway inflammation or asthma.

Obtaining information on other workers who may have developed similar symptoms is also extremely valuable. The physician may have to contact plant officials or local health authorities to obtain this information. It would be most unusual for occupational asthma to be an isolated occurrence. Screening coworkers may help detect other individuals with early manifestations of occupational asthma.

Treating Occupational Asthma

The best treatment for occupational asthma is ending the patient's exposure to the offending agent. This is particularly important because patients can develop chronic asthma, which is not completely reversible. Asthmatic workers may have to change their occupations.

Options other than leaving a job are shifting to activities in the same industry that do not involve exposure to the offending agent, as well as protective clothing or filtration masks. Individuals who are trained in a field and who have developed a unique sensitivity may want to consider immunotherapy. This may be especially helpful for those such as veterinarians who have become sensitized to animal proteins.

Medication therapy should follow the step therapy for mild intermittent, mild persistent, moderate persistent, and severe persistent asthma outlined in Chapter 4. Omalizumab may be particularly helpful in patients with moderate to severe asthma and positive RAST testing for the material that they have been exposed to in the workplace.

A Growing Problem

The occupational asthma problem is likely to get worse as new offending materials are identified in many industries. This affliction may occur in almost any occupation, always manifested by development or worsening of bronchial asthma. The worker often makes the association himself or herself between an offending agent and illness. Once an irritating substance is identified, additional occupational asthma cases are usually discovered.

Remember that occupational asthma is a disease that occurs in the workplace. Outside of work, many asthmatics experience attacks with physical exertion. Chapter 9 discusses the relationship between exercise and asthma.

9

Exercise and Asthma

A PRIMARY GOAL of asthma treatment is maintaining as normal a lifestyle for the patient as possible, including exercise. A large number of children and adults may avoid exercise due to unrecognized asthma. Yet properly managed patients with asthma should be able to pursue exercise as vigorously as anyone. A number of Olympic athletes are asthmatic and have set world records in their events. Many of these individuals endured chest symptoms during competition for months or years before their asthma was diagnosed and effectively treated.

Exercise-Induced Asthma

Considerable research has focused on exercise and asthma. Any person with asthma may experience constriction of the bronchial tubes and worsening of his or her condition when exercising vigorously in cold, dry air. This response has been termed "exercise-induced asthma" (EIA), or "exercise-induced bronchoconstriction" (EIB). EIA probably affects 70 percent to 90 percent of asthmatic patients. In some individuals, particularly children with allergic rhinitis, exercise may be the only trigger for asthma, a phenomenon also noted in adults. These patients only experience asthma with exercise.

How Asthmatics Respond to Exercise

Research has analyzed how people with asthma respond to exercise. During exercise the bronchial tubes remain open as long as asthmatics exercise vigorously. If exercise is stopped abruptly after three to eight minutes, the bronchial tubes tighten and measures of airflow (peak flow and spirometry) show an immediate and progressive decline during the next five to ten minutes. This constriction of the airways may produce wheezing, shortness of breath, chest tightness, and cough, all very similar to an asthma attack triggered by an allergen or other irritant. After twenty to ninety minutes, airflows return to preexercise values.

Why Does Exercise Induce Asthma?

Studies have shown that EIA is probably triggered by a faster exchange of heat and water vapor between the surface lining of the bronchial tubes and inhaled air. It is clear that more vigorous exercise and colder, drier air are more likely to trigger EIA. Any exercise may produce EIA but exercise in cold, dry air produces more intense bronchial spasms. Therefore, extremely sensitive asthma patients should avoid exercising in subfreezing temperatures.

The chemical involved in the rapid constriction of the airways in EIA appears to be a leukotriene. (See Chapter 4.) The improvement noted after the asthma attack appears secondary to the release of a slower acting substance known as a prostaglandin, which acts to relax or dilate the bronchial tubes.

Outdoor exercise may also expose an individual to air pollution and allergens, which have been shown to be triggers of asthmatic attacks. Pollutants also may make susceptible individuals more sensitive to various asthma triggers. As a result, an allergic individual may want to avoid outdoor exercise on high pollen and pollution days.

Making the Diagnosis

Although a diagnosis of EIA may be suspected from a patient's history, doctors may need to perform an exercise test if patients do not manifest asthma any other time. This test may be done with a bicycle ergometer or a treadmill. Spirometry is performed before and after exercise. Patients may also get valuable information by measuring their peak flows before and after exercise.

A young woman recently consulted me after experiencing severe cough after running in New York's Central Park on a cool October day. She had never smoked and was very health conscious, maintaining her ideal weight with a prudent diet. Despite her good health she had always noted that her ability to exercise was less than her peers. She also noted that she was allergic to wheat and frequently had nasal congestion during the allergy months. Her resting pulmonary function tests were normal, but a study performed after a vigorous run revealed constriction of her bronchial tubes, which reversed after the use of a β_2-agonist, confirming EIA. An anti-leukotriene was prescribed, and my patient now notes that she can run distances that previously were unattainable. I wonder if she might have had an athletic career if her EIA had been diagnosed sooner.

It is extremely important to distinguish EIA from other causes of chest symptoms during exercise. These other causes include hardening of the arteries of the heart (atherosclerosis) in which the blood supply to the heart muscle is reduced during exercise, producing chest pain called angina or shortness of breath; illnesses that produce muscle weakness; and exercise-induced closure of the voice box (larynx).

How Should Exercise-Induced Asthma Be Treated?

Treating EIA is preventive. Several agents are effective and are easily adapted for both children and adults.

B_2-Agonists

Short-Acting B_2-Agonists. The short-acting β_2-agonists (see Chapter 4) may be effective in preventing exercise-induced asthma. They are given fifteen minutes before exertion. These agents, however, may not provide sufficient protection in children and adults.

In addition, repeated use may be needed during a day of vigorous exercise.

Long-Acting B$_2$-Agonists. The long-acting β_2-agonists, such as salmeterol and formoterol, provide more protection than the short-acting agents as well as a longer duration of action. In patients who exercise vigorously or are physically active more than once a day, the long-acting agent is preferred. Remember, however, that long-acting β_2-agonists have a slower onset of action and should be given thirty minutes before exercise begins. If asthma symptoms recur after several hours, a second dose should be given.

B$_2$-Agonists for Children. In young children metered-dose inhalers (MDIs) may be difficult to use, so a spacer with or without a face mask may improve delivery of medication. A dry powder inhaler may also be difficult to use. Some children, particularly those younger than age five, may benefit more from a nebulizer that administers the β_2-agonist. Another alternative for young children is the oral syrup form of β_2-agonist taken at least sixty minutes before exercising.

Anti-Leukotrienes. As noted, leukotrienes have been shown to play a central role in EIA. Anti-leukotriene agents (see Chapter 4) have been shown to provide substantial protection against EIA for many patients. These agents also provide several practical advantages. They are taken once daily by mouth and have little adverse effects. Anti-leukotrienes have also been approved for children as young as fifteen months of age. It should be noted that these agents must be maintained on a regular basis to be effective, and it is estimated that they may not be effective in preventing EIA in one out of four patients. Patients who are maintained on anti-leukotriene agents should continue to use their short-acting β_2-agonist on an as-needed basis.

Cromolyn Sodium and Nedocromil Sodium

Cromolyn sodium and nedocromil sodium can also prevent EIA and are an alternative to the β_2-agonists. These agents are given fifteen minutes before exercise. One study comparing cromolyn and albuterol in the prevention of EIA found albuterol more effective.

Theophylline

Theophylline can prevent exercise-induced asthma but is clearly less effective than the β_2-agonists, anti-leukotrienes, cromolyn, and nedocromil.

Inhaled Corticosteroids

Inhaled corticosteroids do not reduce EIA if given as a single dose shortly before exercise. These agents, however, do reduce exercise-induced symptoms if maintained on a regular daily basis.

Approved Medications for Athletes

The NCAA and the International Olympic Committee maintain lists of acceptable medications for athletes. Medications approved by the United States Olympic Committee include β_2-agonists (aerosol forms only) as well as anti-leukotrienes, cromolyn sodium, nedocromil sodium, theophylline, and inhaled corticosteroids.

Guidelines for Preventing Exercise-Induced Asthma

Some simple guidelines are helpful in preventing EIA. First, do not exercise if you have been experiencing frequent attacks or are still recovering from a recent attack. After an attack, consult your physician before embarking on or resuming an exercise program. Second, plan a long warm-up period before and cool-down period after exercise lasting between thirty to sixty minutes. Third, avoid exercise in subfreezing, dry air and wear a face mask or scarf across your nose and face to warm inspired air if you exercise in the cold. Also avoid exercising where the air is polluted such as in areas with heavy traffic. Fourth, discuss your preventive approach to EIA with your physician. If the use of a short-acting β_2-agonist fifteen minutes before exercise is not sufficient in preventing EIA, then either a long-acting β_2-agent or an anti-leukotriene should be added. Table 9.1 summarizes these prevention steps.

If you experience any difficulty with exercise, tell your physician so you can obtain his or her instructions on adjusting your routine. It would help your physician review your case if you obtain peak flow measurements recorded at the time of distress.

How Does Conditioning Affect Asthma?

Recent evidence suggests regular conditioning exercises may have a favorable effect on asthma and the use of medications. Conditioning increases the muscle fitness and improves your body's ability to supply oxygen as fuel. Regular exercise eases breathing effort and increases stamina.

A recent study demonstrated that conditioning of patients with asthma resulted in a greater degree of dilatation of the bronchial

---

Table 9.1   How to Prevent Exercise-Induced Asthma (EIA)

Avoid exercise if your asthma is unstable.

Check with your physician if you are unsure when to start.

Perform a long warm-up and cool down.

Avoid exercise in sub-freezing temperatures.

Always wear a face mask when exercising in cold weather.

Avoid endurance sports.

Avoid outdoor exercise when ozone levels or pollen counts are high.

Use your short-acting β_2-agonist fifteen minutes before exercise.

If EIA Is Not Prevented

Substitute a long-acting β_2-agonist thirty minutes before exercise or a daily anti-leukotriene.

Alternative: Cromolyn or nedocromil one hour before exercise.

Follow step-wise guidelines for persistent asthma.

tubes after exercise, an effect that reduced their potential for EIA. Clearly, if patients follow these guidelines for preventing EIA, they may benefit greatly from regular exercise.

What Type of Exercise Should I Do?

Almost any form of exercise may be undertaken by individuals with asthma. Athletes with asthma have distinguished themselves in many diverse competitions, including swimming, track and field, cycling, and even cross-country skiing. You should find an exercise you enjoy and gradually increase your activity.

Swimming is an ideal exercise for those individuals who are prone to EIA since breathing warm, humid air from a body of water reduces cooling and drying in the bronchial tubes. Swimming in highly chlorinated water, however, increases the risk of developing EIA. It is best to check chlorine levels before swimming and to look for a pool that maintains levels at the low end of the safe range (one to four parts per million). Sports that combine short bursts of activity with periods of rest such as baseball, tennis, sprinting, and volleyball are better than endurance sports such as soccer, basketball, hockey, and long-distance running.

If you are about to start an exercise program, always check first with your physician, who may want you to take an exercise test. Remember, your asthma should be under good control before you start any exercise routine.

You can exercise at home or indoors, especially during the winter months. In fact, indoor exercise may be better for you during high pollen count periods or air pollution alerts. A simple way to begin is with light stretching exercises for the arms, shoulders, and torso. Recent research suggests that conditioning the upper body reduces shortness of breath in many patients with chronic respiratory disease. Upper body exercises may include light weights; some asthmatics prefer weight training to more rigorous programs.

Your exercise regimen will succeed best with regular workouts. You do not have to exercise every day. A routine of twenty to thirty minutes of exercise three times a week is good. Many patients vary their exercises for each workout, increasing their conditioning gradually.

Achieving Your Goal of an Active Lifestyle

For almost all asthmatics, asthma gets worse with exercise; but that fact has not kept individuals with asthma from setting world records in many sports events. Anyone with good control over asthma may begin an exercise program, and the conditioning you achieve may help improve your stamina and reduce shortness of breath. Exercise may also help you reduce stress and anxiety as you build confidence and improve your well-being.

This chapter has offered guidelines and suggestions for developing and performing an asthma exercise regimen, whose benefits are clear. Chapter 10 explores the relationship between asthma and other illnesses that affect the sinuses and the stomach.

10

Asthma and Related Illnesses

ALTHOUGH ASTHMA IS a disease of the lungs, it may be influenced by illnesses that affect other parts of the body. For many asthma patients, treating these related illnesses may even prevent or improve their bronchial asthma condition. Two common examples are disorders of the nose and sinuses and of the digestive tract. This chapter discusses the relationship between asthma and these illnesses.

What Are the Sinuses?

The sinuses are a series of bony cavities located in the skull, lined by a surface layer called the epithelium. This thin membrane closely resembles the bronchial tube lining. Each sinus opens into the nasal passages, which have a similar surface lining. Although this thin surface membrane has a pale, innocent appearance, it may become severely swollen and produce a copious discharge. Figure 10.1 shows the location of the sinuses.

The nasal and sinus passages perform several functions vital to healthy breathing, including filtering air as it is inhaled and trapping foreign particles and germs, as well as warming and adding moisture to inspired air. The importance of the warming function was highlighted in Chapter 9.

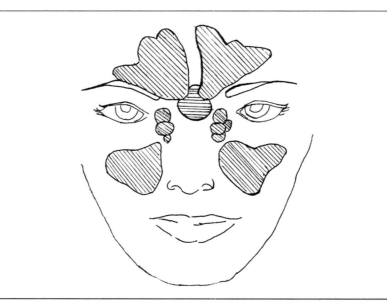

Figure 10.1 The sinuses

Symptoms of Nasal and Sinus Disease

When the lining of the nasal and sinus passages becomes irritated and inflamed, the body's response is similar to what occurs in the bronchial tubes during an asthma attack. This reaction may occur in patients with and without allergies. Swelling of this lining creates congestion and stuffiness. In the nose this inflammation is called rhinitis, and when inflammation occurs too much mucus may be produced, adding to the obstruction. A watery discharge or drip is common with many irritations of the nose and sinuses. Because some of this discharge may be directed back toward the throat, it is often termed "postnasal drip."

In the bony sinuses inhaled germs may take advantage of these wet, warm conditions to produce an infection called sinusitis. When that happens, the back drip may carry disease organisms into the throat and lower respiratory passages. Sinus infections may be slow to resolve and difficult to treat because of lowered blood supply to bony areas. A recent study of sinuses during common colds highlighted the extensive sinus infection and congestion that may exist then. If not adequately treated, sinus disease can become chronic, forming the basis for repeated infections.

How Sinus Disease Can Affect Asthma

Clearly, there is a close relationship between sinus disease and asthma. Patients with active sinus disease may suffer repeated worsening of their asthma. These flare-ups may be partly due to mucus dripping into the throat and windpipe, causing cough and irritation. Infection from the sinuses may also be carried into the lower bronchial tree, triggering inflammation and asthma. This often may occur at night, another reason for nighttime asthma attacks. Nasal and sinus congestion also may produce obstruction of these passages, necessitating mouth breathing, as well as the absence of warming and moisturizing of inhaled air that the nasal and sinus passages produce may also exacerbate bronchial asthma.

How Is Sinusitis Diagnosed?

The characteristic symptoms of sinus disease include nasal congestion, pain, and a discolored mucus discharge. The pain usually occurs above or near the affected sinus. Often, this pain is felt as a severe headache, particularly over the forehead. Facial swelling is also common and so is tenderness above the affected areas. Examination is usually done with a flashlight that looks into the nasal passages, often aided by an instrument called a nasal speculum, which widens the doctor's field of view into the nose. For a more detailed examination with the ability to better visualize the sinus openings, fiber-optic instruments such as the flexible endoscope may be used.

A sinusitis diagnosis may be confirmed by x-ray. Plain sinus films may demonstrate the presence of fluid in the sinus cavities or a thickening of the lining. The more highly detailed computerized axial tomography (CAT) scan is now widely used to diagnose sinusitis because it may pick up disease plain x-ray films miss.

Treating Sinusitis

Antibiotics. The primary treatment for acute sinusitis is antibiotics that eradicate infection. A prolonged course is often needed because the blood supply to bony areas such as the sinuses is limited. This course may vary, but a typical treatment takes three weeks.

Establishing Drainage. In sinus disease it is crucial to establish good drainage, which is often achieved with decongestants such as pseudoephedrine. A second-generation antihistamine can also help, particularly in allergic patients. To avoid excessive dryness, decongestants are often combined with an expectorant such as guaifenesin. Guaifenesin may also be taken without decongestant and is available in liquid (Robitussin Expectorant) or tablet (Mucinex) form without prescription. A saline nasal spray should be used to help rinse out dried secretions and add moisture to dry membranes.

Treating Chronic Sinusitis

Even after a sinus infection has been eradicated, many patients will continue to experience congestion, pain, and recurring bouts of sinus infection. In patients with chronic disease, particularly allergic ones, adding intranasal corticosteroid sprays may be extremely helpful in reducing inflammation. Beclomethasone (Vancenase), budesonide (Rhinocort Aqua), fluticasone (Flonase), flunisolide (Nasarel), mometasone (Nasonex), and triamcinolone (Nasacort Aqua) are available in the United States. Intranasal cromolyn sodium (Nasalcrom) may also help these patients.

Should You Consider Surgery?

In patients who suffer from persistent sinus infections despite courses of appropriate antibiotics, a surgical drainage procedure may be needed. A sinus CAT scan documenting the presence of infection and maximal medical therapy should be given before surgery. This surgery is increasingly performed through the endoscope. The technique is less traumatic than older sinus drainage procedures and is often performed in an outpatient setting.

Physicians must individualize treatment of sinus disease for each patient. Aggressive treatment of sinus disease, however, may also improve the control of bronchial asthma.

What Is Rhinitis?

Rhinitis is inflammation of the nasal membranes. Allergic rhinitis occurs when a sensitive individual is exposed to allergens such as pollens, mold, and dust mites. This may be seasonal as in the individual who is sensitive to ragweed (hay fever) and becomes symptomatic in August and September. Allergic rhinitis may occur year-round (perennial) in persons who are sensitive to animal dander, dust, or other indoor allergens. In addition, rhinitis may be nonallergic in which inflammation occurs without allergy (also called vasomotor rhinitis). Nonallergic rhinitis is typically due to exposure to cigarette smoke or other pollutants.

Rhinitis and Asthma: Is There a Link?

Recent research has established a definite link between allergic rhinitis and asthma. Some investigators have referred to these two entities as "united airways disease" since the nerve and blood supply and lining of the nose and bronchial tubes are very similar. In addition, the nose acts as a filter, heat exchanger, and humidifier for inhaled air. If the nasal passages fail to provide these functions, the lower airways of the lung are greatly affected. The body cells and chemical mediators that produce inflammation in the nose are also similar to those found in the bronchial tubes of people with asthma.

Based on this information it is not surprising that one report estimated that up to 78 percent of patients with asthma have nasal symptoms and 38 percent of patients with allergic rhinitis have asthma. Further reports have suggested that aggressive control of rhinitis may prevent the development of asthma in some individuals. In many others, the treatment of rhinitis has been found to be an essential part of an asthma control treatment program.

Treating Allergic Rhinitis

Treating allergic rhinitis in many ways is similar to treating sinusitis. Second-generation antihistamines with or without decongestants may be prescribed for patients with bronchial asthma without adverse effects. Intranasal topical corticosteroid sprays and cromolyn sodium are extremely helpful in treating rhinitis. These agents do not produce excessive dryness and may be preferred in some patients over antihistamines and decongestants. Adverse effects of topical corticosteroid nasal sprays include minor irritation or stinging and bleeding from the nasal lining. A saline nasal mist or gel can help provide moisture to the nasal passages.

Anti-leukotrienes have also been approved for the treatment of allergic rhinitis and have the double effect of being both "anti-allergy" and "anti-asthma." They are usually given to individuals with allergic rhinitis when trials of antihistamines and intranasal corticosteroids have not been effective.

Allergy injections or immunotherapy continue to be an option for people with allergic rhinitis. Compared to the treatments already noted, they are more time-consuming and require an extended period before they become effective.

What Are Nasal Polyps?

Nasal polyps are fleshy growths or extensions of the nasal and sinus lining. They are common in patients with bronchial asthma and may occur with or without allergy. They often occur in patients older than age forty who are not allergic but who have severe rhinitis. Common symptoms are constant nasal stuffiness as well as a loss or reduction of the senses of smell and/or taste.

The importance of nasal polyps is related to their ability to block the nasal and sinus passages, which may also be the source of poor drainage of sinuses that leads to recurring sinus infections. The presence of nasal polyps in adult patients who are not allergic often identifies a more severe group of asthmatics. This group also has a greater hypersensitivity to aspirin and related medications (see Chapter 11).

Treating Nasal Polyps

Administering topical intranasal corticosteroid sprays often helps nasal polyps. Oral corticosteroids may be used to shrink polyps in patients with severe disease. In those who do not respond and who have severe obstructions, polypectomy should be considered. When feasible, this procedure is performed endoscopically. Before polypectomy occurs, the patient's asthma must be under good control, which may demand pretreatment with oral corticosteroids. Unfortunately, polyps tend to recur.

Asthma and the Stomach

More and more clearly there seems to be some relationship between bronchial asthma and stomach function. Asthmatics often suffer from digestive problems, frequently complaining about excess stomach acid. As a result, treating stomach disorders may actually improve the control of unstable asthmatics who are prone to frequent attacks.

The Esophagus

The human digestive tract includes a feeding passage known as the esophagus through which food passes before entering the stomach to begin digestion. The esophagus is in the chest just behind the windpipe and starts at about the same level as the voice box (larynx). At the lower end of the esophagus a muscular ring, or sphincter, that relaxes to open and tightens to close ensures stomach contents remain in the stomach where they are exposed to acid. In many digestive disorders the esophageal sphincter may malfunction, allowing a reflux of acid back into the esophagus. This is called gastroesophageal reflux disease (GERD). Increasing evidence suggests this disorder is related to reduced motion or motility of the feeding passage and stomach. An associated condition is overproduction of acid or hyperacidity. A common contributing condition to GERD is a hiatal hernia, in which a fold of the stomach lining protrudes upward into the esophagus.

Asthma and Reflux

Research shows a high incidence of gastroesophageal reflux in patients with bronchial asthma. It is unclear how much of a contributing factor GERD is to bronchial asthma since many studies have resulted in conflicting conclusions. Also unclear is how acid reflux aggravates bronchial asthma. In rare cases the actual aspiration of acid into the bronchial tubes may occur, producing severe inflammation. The mere presence of acid in the esophagus may even trigger a reflex leading to bronchoconstriction. Despite the conflicting study conclusions, some patients with GERD and asthma have benefited from the treatment of reflux, which has reduced the frequency of their asthma attacks.

Asthma Medications That May Aggravate Stomach Disorders

Several asthma medications may irritate your stomach. Oral corticosteroids may produce gastritis as well as ulceration of the stomach lining. Theophylline may irritate the stomach lining, causing gastritis. In patients with preexisting hyperacidity, theophylline and oral corticosteroids may aggravate their conditions and increase reflux.

When Should You Suspect Gastroesophageal Reflux?

In many asthma patients, the symptoms of gastroesophageal reflux may be obvious, including heartburn and belching, complaints most apparent after meals and during sleep when the person is reclining. Other patients, however, are entirely without symptoms. Examining the voice box may reveal telltale signs of acid irritation. Further proof of reflux may be obtained through endoscopic examination of the esophagus as well as through x-rays of the upper digestive tract. Asthma attacks often occur at night, so it may be unclear whether an attack is related to reflux. A distinguishing feature of GERD-related asthma may be the patient's inability to prevent nighttime attacks despite maximal asthma therapy.

Treating Gastroesophageal Reflux

Patients may reduce reflux by not eating at least two hours before bedtime and by elevating the head of their beds by six to eight inches. Patients should avoid alcohol, caffeine, and highly seasoned foods. Medications such as theophylline and oral corticosteroids may need to be reduced or eliminated in patients who do not respond to medical measures for controlling reflux.

Many medications can be used to treat reflux. These medications should only be used as directed by your physician. Too many patients overuse antacids trying to reduce heartburn. Your physician may prescribe one of two groups of medications that reduce stomach acid, either an H2 antagonist such as famotidine (Pepcid) or a stronger proton pump inhibitor such as omeprazole (Prilosec). Antacids may be used to supplement these medications in patients with severe reflux. Studies of patients with asthma and reflux who were treated with these agents have shown improvement in their asthmatic condition.

Your physician also may prescribe a medication that increases esophagus motility and emptying of the stomach, thus reducing reflux. Called prokinetic agents, these medications are taken before meals and at bedtime. Metoclopramide (Reglan) is the only prokinetic agent available in the United States. It has been found to have significant adverse effects such as drowsiness.

In rare instances medical therapy may fail and surgical treatment should be considered. This procedure has been performed with a less invasive laparoscopic approach in which the surgeon operates through a small opening in the belly using video guidance.

Aggressively treating gastroesophageal reflux in patients with uncontrolled asthma may successfully reduce the frequency of asthma attacks. This condition should be searched out in patients whose asthma is difficult to control despite maximal therapy.

Conclusion: Look for Related Illnesses

Asthma and illnesses may affect the nose and sinuses and digestive tract. Patients who have unstable asthma should look outside their chests to spot aggravating factors such as sinusitis, rhinitis, and reflux of stomach acid. For many patients, identifying and treating these related illnesses may improve their bronchial asthma condition.

11

Asthma and Special Considerations

ASTHMA MAY BE thought of as oversensitivity to a variety of stimuli or circumstances that may trigger an attack. These include reactions to certain medications such as aspirin, changes in hormone levels, changes in sleep, and the stresses of surgery. Asthma attacks may be prevented by preparing for special situations, such as surgery, or by being aware of potential triggers.

Asthma and Surgery

Surgery may present several problems for asthmatics and must be approached carefully. To avoid complications there should be close communication prior to the procedure between the surgeon and the physician responsible for managing the patient's asthma.

Possible Complications

Complications may arise from several sources in patients with asthma who undergo surgery. When general anesthesia is required, the windpipe is intubated with a tube connected to a respirator. Under anesthesia, the respirator provides mechanical breathing and ensures the exchange of oxygen and carbon dioxide. In asthma patients, intubating the windpipe may trigger reflexes originating in the throat that can lead to bronchoconstriction. Therefore, alternatives to general anesthesia—local, regional, and spinal—should always be considered, depending greatly upon the type of surgery and the surgeon's preference.

Further complications may be caused by bronchoconstriction during and after surgery. Oxygen and carbon dioxide levels may be affected. Surgery is often a source of decreased depth of breathing; as a result, the small air sacs of the lung may collapse, a condition known as atelectasis. This condition may also lower oxygen levels and, combined with the presence of bronchoconstriction, can produce an even greater drop in blood oxygen. More severe atelectasis can be expected in patients who undergo general anesthesia. Thick bronchial mucus of asthma may clog airways and increase the risk of lung infection.

Complications vary greatly depending on the surgery performed. The greatest risk occurs from procedures involving the chest, such as heart or lung operations. Surgery performed on the upper abdomen, such as gall bladder removal, may also impact lung function significantly.

How to Avoid Complications from Surgery

With careful preparation that identifies patients at greater risk, surgical complications can be avoided. For instance, newer anesthesia techniques that avoid intubation are one way to prevent serious complications. Even in the mildest asthmatic patient, preparation is needed before surgery.

The Preoperative Evaluation. If surgery is needed, a preoperative evaluation should be performed by the primary physician, even in patients who are under good control, because complications may arise in any asthmatic patient. Patients with moderate to severe asthma are certainly at greater risk for complications and should have diligent preoperative checkups.

During the preoperative evaluation, the patient's history, medications, and flow rates or spirometry should be reviewed. The frequency of asthma attacks should be noted as well as the person's need for bronchodilator sprays and corticosteroids.

Allergies to medications and previous reactions to anesthesia also should be noted at this time. The patient should be instructed on how to take asthma medication before surgery, since many procedures are now performed outpatient or the same day.

When Surgery Should Be Postponed. Patients undergoing elective surgery whose asthma is not under good control should postpone their procedures to allow proper administration of medication. In emergencies, this delay may not be possible, so asthma therapy may have to be given intravenously during and after surgery.

Preparing for Surgery

Preparing for surgery may include a course of oral corticosteroids in patients who are symptomatic or who show significant reductions in flow rates on spirometry. In stable patients the medication regimen should continue right up to the time of surgery. To avoid reflex bronchoconstriction, β_2-agonists may be given by inhalation just before surgery. Because all oral intake is usually stopped for several hours before surgery, patients receiving theophylline may be affected, although long-acting preparations may maintain blood levels for up to twelve hours. In patients who must maintain a therapeutic blood level for good control of their asthma, intravenous aminophylline may ensure a constant level.

Patients with moderate to severe asthma who have required daily doses or frequent courses of oral corticosteroids should receive intravenous injections of corticosteroids at the time of surgery to prevent exacerbation of their conditions and possible adrenal insufficiency. Steroids should also be given in the postoperative period. Inhalation therapy with bronchodilators such as β_2-agonists and anticholinergic medication should also be continued after surgery.

After Surgery

Once the asthma patient has stabilized after surgery, an attempt should be made to resume the patient's maintenance asthma medication as soon as possible. In patients whose asthma has worsened, an oral steroid course may be given with a gradual lowering of the dosage.

Aspirin-Induced Asthma

Allergy to aspirin and related medications may trigger asthmatic attacks in as many as 20 percent of adult asthmatics. This sensitivity appears to be more common in severe adult asthmatics, especially those who have nasal polyps and sinusitis. These patients are also often steroid dependent. However, this reaction may occur in any asthmatic patient, although it is rare in children. The cause of this reaction appears to be related to inhibition by aspirin of the enzyme cyclooxygenase-1 (COX-1), which is followed by overproduction of leukotrienes. (See Chapter 4.) A large group of medications that also produce this inhibition, the nonsteroidal anti-inflammatory drugs (NSAIDs), may cause the same asthmatic reaction, too.

Recent research suggests that there are other pathways involved in aspirin-induced asthma (AIA) since the above mechanism does not explain why aspirin does not cause asthma in all individuals.

Characteristic Features of Aspirin-Induced Asthma

The most common presentation of AIA is an adult patient who first develops severe nasal symptoms of congestion and drip. Sinusitis may also develop and nasal polyps are often discovered on examination. In these patients, bronchial asthma may not be present at first but tends to develop after the nasal problems. Once asthma surfaces, it is often severe and unstable.

Several characteristics of AIA should be emphasized. Aspirin may produce an asthmatic attack even in patients who have previously taken it without any reaction. These attacks are usually severe, occurring within one hour of aspirin ingestion. The reaction may include flushing, nasal congestion, and eye irritation in addition to the asthmatic attack. Even a single aspirin tablet (or other anti-inflammatory agent that may cause bronchoconstriction) may produce a potentially fatal asthma attack. Once sensitivity to aspirin is established it does not resolve, and asthma patients should never again take this medication.

How the Diagnosis Is Made

The definitive diagnosis of AIA may only be made by documenting a reaction to this medication. A challenge test may be performed by experienced physicians with immediate access to medication to counter a severe reaction. Documentation may also be made through an accurate medical history. If so, the physician may not feel a challenge test is needed. Because of the danger of developing a severe asthma attack from aspirin ingestion, all asthma patients should avoid using aspirin.

Treatment of Choice

Leukotrienes have been found to be highly active in patients with aspirin-induced asthma. These chemicals appear to be the most important mediators of the asthmatic response in patients with aspirin-induced asthma. Treatment with an anti-leukotriene agent (zileuton, zafirlukast, or montelukast) has been highly effective in controlling asthmatic attacks in these patients.

Nonsteroidal Anti-Inflammatory Drugs

Nonsteroidal anti-inflammatory drugs that inhibit the enzyme cyclooxygenase may also cause a severe asthma reaction. For a partial list of these drugs see Table 11.1. Many new NSAIDs are being introduced that are widely prescribed for pain, headache, joint disease, and menstrual cramps. Two NSAIDs, ibuprofen and naproxen, are available without prescription. Aspirin and ibuprofen also are often included in cold remedies sold over the counter. Patients should carefully review the ingredients of any over-the-counter medication and if unsure of its safety, consult their physician. Generally, you should avoid "cold pills" since they often combine aspirin and first-generation antihistamines, two agents that may produce adverse reactions in patients with bronchial asthma.

*Table 11.1   Medications That May Produce Asthma in
Aspirin-Sensitive Patients**

Drug Name	Brand Name
Aspirin	Empirin, Fiorinal, Percodan, Equagesic, Ecotrin**
Diclofenac	Voltaren
Diflunisal	Dolobid
Fenoprofen	Nalfon
Ketoprofen	Orudis
Flurbiprofen	Ansaid
Ibuprofen	Advil, Motrin, Nuprin
Indomethacin	Indocin
Mefenamic Acid	Ponstel
Meloxicam	Mobic
Naproxen	Aleve, Anaprox, Naprosyn
Oxaprozin	Daypro
Piroxicam	Feldene
Sulfinpyrazone	Anturane
Sulindac	Clinoril
Tolmetin	Tolectin

*This is only a partial list.

**Many over-the-counter medications contain aspirin and are not listed.

Because of possible asthmatic reactions to NSAIDs, patients with asthma should in general avoid these medications. In patients with illnesses such as rheumatoid arthritis where these medications are often needed, however, physicians may feel that a trial of an NSAID under close observation is indicated. As an alternative, anti-inflammatory medications that do not inhibit cyclooxygenase-1 (COX-1) may be tried.

Nonsteroidal anti-inflammatory drugs that inhibit cyclooxygenase-2 (COX-2), such as rofecoxib (Vioxx) and celecoxib (Celebrex), were introduced several years ago but have been the source of considerable controversy in regard to adverse cardiovascular side effects. Celecoxib is the only COX-2 inhibitor still available in the United States. Studies of patients with asthma and aspirin allergy have found that COX-2 inhibitors are a safe alternative for treatment of inflammatory conditions.

Additional alternatives to aspirin and NSAIDs include acetaminophen, sodium thiosalicylate, and choline magnesium trisalicylate. Acetaminophen, widely available without prescription, has reportedly produced asthma attacks in a small number of patients. This reaction is extremely rare and as a rule, this drug represents a safe alternative to aspirin and the NSAIDs, but it lacks anti-inflammatory properties. Sodium thiosalicylate and choline magnesium trisalicylate are anti-inflammatory drugs that do not inhibit cyclooxygenase and are safe alternatives to aspirin and NSAIDs. These medications are only available by prescription.

Nocturnal Asthma

Nighttime can be an extremely difficult period for individuals with bronchial asthma. All asthma patients have more sensitive airways at night. Those with increased attacks at night, "nocturnal asthma," have been found to experience an eightfold increase in airway hyperreactivity. Remember, the presence of nocturnal attacks is one of the factors that differentiates mild from moderate and severe asthmatics.

Adding to the significance of nocturnal asthma is increasing data that fatal attacks are more common at night. Several studies show a greater incidence of severe and fatal attacks between midnight and 8 a.m. These data have prompted greater investigation into the source and treatment of nocturnal asthma.

What Causes Nocturnal Asthma?

At one time it was thought nocturnal asthma was caused by the "wearing off" of medication during the night. Further research has shown that there is an exaggerated narrowing of the airways during nocturnal and early morning asthma. Several factors appear to be involved.

Adrenal Connection. It is well documented that there is a natural rhythm of the body in which many organs function differently during the night. The adrenal gland is no exception. During sleep the adrenal gland manufactures less cortisone and epinephrine, causing a drop in their blood levels. Both of these substances are protective against asthma and promote bronchial dilatation so that this dip in blood levels may be one explanation for nocturnal asthma attacks.

The Environment. Patients suffering nocturnal asthmatic attacks should look carefully at their bedrooms for sources of irritation. Potential allergens commonly found in bedrooms include feather pillows, animal dander, and dust mites. Simply using pillow and mattress covers may dramatically reduce nocturnal attacks. Other steps for removing allergens are detailed in Chapter 6.

Reflux Connection. In Chapter 10 the relationship between asthma and the stomach was discussed. Some doctors believe some nocturnal asthmatic attacks may be caused by reflux of stomach acid into the esophagus and throat, where it may be aspirated into the bronchial tubes. Aggressive treatment of gastroesophageal reflux may reduce the frequency of nocturnal attacks.

Sinusitis and Nocturnal Asthma. The relationship between asthma and sinusitis was also discussed in Chapter 10. Animal studies suggest that aspirating infected material from the sinuses into the lower throat and bronchial tubes may produce nocturnal asthma attacks. Although this effect has yet to be proven in patients with asthma, the strong possibility of a connection should reinforce vigorous treatment of sinusitis.

Other Factors. Other factors may play a role in nocturnal asthma. It appears there is some cooling of airways at night. In asthmatics this change in temperature may be enough to produce asthma attacks. This mechanism also plays a role in exercise-induced asthma.

In addition, some element in the nervous system may be more active at night. The vagus nerve in the cholinergic nervous system is more active at night, and an increase in vagal tone may constrict the bronchial airways. In asthma patients that constriction may increase the frequency of attacks.

Treating Nocturnal Asthma

Treating nocturnal asthma is based on the goal of achieving sufficient medication levels during sleep hours as well as eliminating environmental allergens. However, studies have shown that if patients are well controlled during the day, they will experience fewer and/or milder attacks at night. Asthma should always be regarded as a twenty-four-hour illness, and treatment should not be directed solely at the nighttime hours.

Choosing Medication for Nocturnal Asthma. Many medications may be used to treat nocturnal asthma, and more than one agent may be needed for patients with severe and frequent attacks.

B_2-agonists are available in long-acting forms both in aerosol (salmeterol or formoterol) and tablet form (albuterol) that may be administered at night. By improving lung function and preventing nocturnal attacks, these agents may actually improve quality of sleep.

In sustained-release forms, theophylline allows once- or twice-a-day dosing and is suitable for nocturnal asthma treatment. The physician can time administration of this medication so peak blood levels are obtained during sleep. A common approach is one sustained-release preparation after the evening meal. Remember, theophylline blood levels can be measured and each sustained-release preparation is unique. One drawback of theophylline for nocturnal asthma is its potentially adverse side effect of insomnia. Patients who limit their caffeine intake may reduce this effect.

Because overactivity of the cholinergic nervous system has been implicated in nocturnal asthma, anticholingeric agents have been administered at bedtime in patients with nocturnal asthma. High doses (ten puffs) of ipratropium bromide have been administered with conflicting results in several studies. At this time it does not appear that this agent is more effective than long-acting B_2-agonists for treating nocturnal asthma.

Patients with moderate to severe nocturnal asthma may need oral corticosteroids to control their symptoms. Studies of the timing of administration of this medication have shown dosing in early morning or evening does not achieve better control of nocturnal asthma. In these studies, patients who took steroid dosages at 3 p.m., however, significantly reduced the likelihood of nocturnal attacks.

Patients who continue to suffer nocturnal attacks despite aggressive therapy may need to awaken one hour before their usual nighttime attack to administer a short-acting β_2-agonist, an approach termed "therapeutic awakening."

Antidepressant Medication and B-Agonists

Monoamine oxidase (MAO) inhibitors are commonly prescribed for depression. These drugs inhibit the enzyme responsible for breaking down epinephrine released from the adrenal gland. When a β-adrenergic agonist is administered to patients receiving an MAO inhibitor, there is a greater risk of adverse effects on the circulation, such as blood pressure elevation. This is more likely when the β-agonist is given by mouth or by injection since there is higher total-body absorption of the drug. By inhaling a β-agonist, there is less chance of producing an adverse effect in a patient receiving an MAO inhibitor. When possible, an alternative antidepressant should be substituted in asthma patients to permit safe administration of a β-agonist. Patients who must receive both medications should be monitored closely for adverse circulatory effects.

Sedatives and Asthma

In asthma, as in other chronic illnesses, patients may experience increased levels of anxiety as well as sleeplessness. Requests for tranquilizers and sleeping pills are common. In patients with severe asthma, shortness of breath and fear of hospitalization may further heighten anxiety levels. Sleep may also be interrupted by asthmatic attacks.

Why to Avoid Tranquilizers and Sleeping Pills

All tranquilizers and sleeping pills affect the brain center that drives breathing. This reduces the activity of this vital center and causes more shallow breaths. Shallow breathing does not produce full expansion of the lung and results in lower oxygen levels. In patients with severe asthma, tranquilizers and sedatives may depress breathing, which worsens attacks, with possible life-threatening results. These patients should always avoid these agents.

Exceptions to the Rule

Patients with mild asthma and anxiety disorders such as panic attacks that require medication may receive tranquilizers. In these patients, close communication must be established between the primary physician and the psychiatrist prescribing the anxiety medication to ensure proper monitoring. This should include spirometry and a careful record of peak flows. Sleeping pills should generally be avoided even in patients with mild asthma other than for short-term use and only under careful physician supervision.

Oxygen Use in Asthma

When treating bronchial asthma, oxygen should be confined mainly to the emergency room and hospital setting because only in severe attacks do oxygen levels drop significantly. Besides, oxygen will not relieve bronchial constriction or in any way shorten an asthma attack.

There are some exceptions to this rule. Patients who have had severe, rapidly developing attacks in the past with low oxygen levels noted on admission to the hospital and who are difficult to control may keep an emergency oxygen cylinder at home. Patients with bronchial asthma and associated conditions such as congestive heart failure or other heart diseases who might not tolerate any drop in oxygen level may also keep a home emergency oxygen supply. Avoid routine use of oxygen in the home to treat uncomplicated bronchial asthma.

Premenstrual Asthma

Premenstrual asthma is common, affecting 40 percent to 100 percent of female asthmatics. Severe asthma attacks appear to be more common in the premenstrual phase. Studies have demonstrated heightened sensitivity to various asthma triggers before menstruation. A further report revealed that premenopausal women are most likely to suffer an asthma attack in the premenstrual phase of the menstrual cycle when estrogen levels are lowest. Hormonal treatment has been given to patients who suffer severe premenstrual exacerbations of their asthma. This has included the use of progesterone, estrogen, and gonadotrophin-releasing hormone analogues, which induce a reversible menopause. Additional measures that are helpful involve a step-by-step increase in medication, possibly including a premenstrual increase in inhaled corticosteroid or a brief course of oral corticosteroid.

Just as in pregnancy, asthma varies from patient to patient prior to menstruation. Recording peak flows should help identify this form of asthma.

Menopause and Asthma

After menopause, the relationship between asthma and estrogen is less clear. Postmenopausal women who have not taken hormone replacement therapy appear to have a lower risk of asthma than premenopausal women. Postmenopausal women who have taken or continue to take hormone replacement therapy have been found to have an increased risk of developing asthma. In addition, the risk of asthma appears to increase with higher doses of hormone replacement.

Sex and Asthma

The goal of achieving a normal lifestyle despite the presence of bronchial asthma certainly includes sexual activity. Sex should be regarded as healthy exercise to which many of the precautions concerning exercise-induced asthma can be applied.

Asthma medications do not affect sexual performance and can prevent asthmatic attacks that may be triggered by sexual activity. B-agonists should be taken prior to sex and cromolyn or nedocromil may be added if the β-agonist proves ineffective. Be sure you allow enough time for the medication to take effect. Avoiding allergens in the bedroom may be particularly important for sensitive patients to prevent attacks during sexual activity. Be sure to follow the steps for reducing dust mites in pillows, mattresses, and bed covers. Perfumes or colognes also may trigger attacks and should be avoided.

Patients and their sexual partners may want to discuss with their physicians problems they have encountered during sex. Some patients may be more comfortable using positions that do not cause pressure to the chest. If asthma attacks have occurred during sex, reassurance to allay anxiety and additional steps to avoid further attacks should be discussed with physicians.

Asthma and Work Disability

Asthma is a frequent cause of work disability. In adults between the ages of eighteen and forty-four, asthma is second only to back problems as the leading cause of medical absence from work. A recent study of disability among adult asthmatics revealed that asthma frequently results in changes in jobs and work duties that may cause a reduction in income.

How Is Work Disability Determined?

The variable nature of bronchial asthma makes determining a work disability extremely difficult. Criteria for disability related to pulmonary disorders are based on measurements of lung function through pulmonary function tests. Patients with severe asthma may have symptom-free periods when lung function measurements exceed the criteria set by the American Medical Association.

Therefore, it is important to consider the frequency of your asthma attacks, what medications you need to control symptoms. and any reduction in day-to-day activities if you're being considered for work disability.

One important characteristic often present in patients disabled from bronchial asthma is dependence on oral corticosteroids to control their disease. Work-disabled patients are often symptomatic despite maximum therapy with medication and are extremely limited in their activities. At least one study of disability in adult asthmatics has found a better correlation between disability and patient symptoms and the medications they need than with pulmonary function results. Guidelines combining all these factors need to be developed to better define disability in bronchial asthma.

Asthma and Pneumonia

A recent report has revealed an increased risk of bacterial pneumonia in asthmatics, age two to forty-nine. The study revealed that this group of asthmatics had almost twice the risk of developing pneumonia due to *Streptococcus pneumoniae* than a comparable group of nonasthmatics.

Streptococcus pneumoniae ("pneumococcus") is the most common cause of bacterial pneumonia. A vaccine against pneumococcal pneumonia (Pneumovax) is recommended for individuals age fifty or older and for high-risk groups, including patients with heart disease, diabetes, and chronic obstructive pulmonary disease (COPD). Further studies are needed to determine if asthma should be added to this list.

12

Asthma and Alternative Medicine

A RECENT STUDY concluded that nearly one-third of the English-speaking population in the United States may utilize unconventional therapy. In non-English-speaking patients living in this country, the use of alternative choices to conventional therapy is higher. Despite further scientific advances in the understanding of asthma, many asthmatics choose alternative forms of treatment. Patients who choose unorthodox forms of treatment often lack faith in modern medicine or are deterred by the way it is practiced.

Unfortunately, some of the alternative forms of treatment may be detrimental. These treatments have not been subjected to the vigorous scientific scrutiny that new asthma medications must undergo before their release. Researchers have recently found that adult asthmatics using herbs were at 2.5 times the risk for asthma hospitalization compared with asthma sufferers not using herbs. Coffee or black tea use was associated with a tripled risk compared with asthmatics not using these beverages for self-treatment.

Many forms of alternative medicine such as changes in lifestyle can be used to complement traditional treatment. Before pursuing any alternative therapy, patients should always consult with their physicians.

What Are the Alternatives?

The major alternative therapies are dietary and lifestyle modifications, herbal medicines, indigenous practices such as Chinese medicine, relaxation therapy, chiropractic care, and pseudoscientific practices. Each of these alternatives has attracted large numbers of followers despite the absence of proven benefits from many of these practices.

"I'm Drinking Black Tea"

L.T. is a sixty-six-year-old CEO of a major company who has been under my care for several years. He is usually seen on an emergency basis, often after a lapse of more than a year. When he is seen, he is usually wheezing and requires corticosteroids to avoid hospitalization. I have prescribed a regimen of a short-acting β_2-agonist and a topical corticosteroid spray. With each exacerbation, I have explained the basis of treatment as well as possible adverse effects. On his last emergency visit I asked if he was following my directions and he said that he was not. The patient explained that he was afraid of possible side effects and had chosen Chinese medicine. "I am drinking black tea," he said. When I asked what was in it, he replied, "I don't know." When I asked why he chose an unknown remedy that might be harmful over a medication that had gone through extensive testing, he replied, "I just don't like to take medicine."

Unfortunately, many intelligent patients choose similar remedies over traditional medicine. After another severe attack that required a night in an emergency room for treatment, the CEO is now using his steroid spray.

Stress and Asthma

Research has shown that anxiety, depression, and other forms of psychological stress may worsen asthma and allergies. One study pinpointed an adverse effect of stress on the immune system. An association between maternal stress and infant wheezing has also been documented.

Based on this information, it is clear that stress management techniques (biofeedback and counseling) may have a beneficial effect on asthma control. One study that had patients with asthma write about their stressful experiences showed a significant positive effect.

Changes in Lifestyle

Lifestyle change as alternative treatment is often called holistic therapy and includes breathing exercises, chiropractic care, and diet.

Breathing Exercises. Breathing exercises that focus on the use of abdominal or belly muscles have been helpful for relaxation and the reduction of anxiety. Many patients have found benefits in yoga or Chinese tai-chi.

Chiropractic Care. Chiropractic care has grown in this country with its application to many conditions, including asthma. Many anecdotal reports from chiropractors and their patients have suggested benefits from this therapy. Three randomized, controlled trials of chiropractic care for asthma, however, have shown that manual therapy does not significantly alter pulmonary function tests, peak flows, or other measures of asthma severity.

Diet. Considerable research into the role of diet and asthma (see Chapter 6) has failed to produce definite conclusions as to the benefit of specific nutrients and supplements. Changes in diet that allow loss of excessive weight, however, may be helpful in reducing shortness of breath.

Vitamins. Vitamin C has been extensively investigated with conflicting results. A recent randomized, controlled study concluded that vitamin C had no effect on asthma control. When given in combination with other antioxidants, however, vitamin C appeared to offer some protection against asthmatic attacks.

Vitamin E has not been studied extensively in asthma but evidence to date would indicate no definite benefit. Vitamin A and a food extract rich in the carotenoid lycopene appeared to protect against exercise-induced asthma in two research studies.

A recent study has suggested that vitamin D may help people with severe asthma who fail to respond to corticosteroids. This supplement may potentially be used to reduce the amount of steroid needed for asthma control.

Minerals. As noted in Chapter 6, a diet high in magnesium may be helpful in controlling asthma. In addition, magnesium has been given intravenously to individuals with severe acute asthmatic attacks with some benefit.

There is conflicting information on the value of selenium, copper, zinc, and other minerals in asthma. As a result, the role of these nutrients is unclear.

Fatty Acids. In some reports when taken in high doses, omega-3 polyunsaturated fatty acids from fish oils has provided some protection against asthma and allergy. Studies of omega-6 and trans-fatty acids, however, have demonstrated an increased risk of asthma.

Probiotics. Probiotics are cultures of potentially beneficial bacteria that normally reside in the healthy intestine. Probiotic-supplemented yogurt consumption has resulted in reduced inflammation and allergic symptoms in some individuals, but one study found no effect on asthma symptoms and lung function.

Chinese Medicine

Many asthmatics have sought help through Chinese medicine. One of the most common treatments is acupuncture. This ancient form of therapy is of little value in an acute asthmatic attack. Some mild benefit in the control of chronic asthma has been reported by individual patients, but further study is needed.

Chinese herbal preparations usually include ephedrine (ma huang), which is a less effective bronchodilator than the β_2-adrenergic agonists. This stimulant may have significant adverse effects (tremors, insomnia, and palpitations) and should be avoided. Large doses of ephedrine may also produce urinary hesitation and occasionally the inability to urinate. Gingko extracts and other herbal remedies such as forskolin have little value in asthma. A traditional form of Chinese medicine called kanpo is popular in Japan but has no proven benefit in asthma.

Western Herbal Remedies

Although a number of asthma drugs such as cromolyn (khella) have evolved from herbal sources, there are no American or European herbs that are of proven value in the treatment of asthma. A number of herbs such as coltsfoot, mullein, hyssop, and elecampine have been recommended by herbalists but do not appear to relieve asthma. These agents do have an effect on the mobilization of mucus and help patients expectorate excess secretions, which may account for the improvement noted by some asthmatics.

Pseudoscience

A number of bizarre remedies with no scientific value have been advocated for the treatment of asthma. These include the administration of hydrogen peroxide, magnetic healing, chelation, and crystal therapy. Patients must be alert to fraudulent practices such as alternative drug preparations, which may actually contain potent corticosteroids.

Why Alternative Therapies May Appear to Work

It has been established that measurable health benefits can occur from an inactive agent (placebo) that patients take in the belief that it may be helpful. A significant placebo response, which may equal that of a proven drug, may occur in at least 30 percent of asthmatics. A "reverse placebo effect" in which asthmatics developed bronchospasm when they were given a bronchodilator (which they were told was a bronchoconstrictor) has also been documented.

In view of this high degree of suggestibility, it is not surprising that many alternative therapies can produce a subjective improvement in asthma, especially when the patient is a strong advocate of a particular discipline or treatment.

Choosing the Proper Therapy

The traditional treatment of asthma has been the combination of avoidance of asthma triggers and a medication regimen that is constructed for each individual patient. A recent scientific symposium supported the use of complementary or alternative medicine in the management of allergy and asthma. The symposium also concluded that the safety of alternative forms of treatment, particularly herbal therapies, was a concern.

Patients should consult with their physicians before beginning any unorthodox form of therapy. In some instances, such as stress management, changes in diet, and breathing exercises, alternative therapies may be used to supplement traditional medicine.

13

Future Considerations

FURTHER ADVANCES IN understanding the genetics and mechanisms of asthma will allow future treatments to be targeted to the individual, permitting better responses to treatment. Scientists have already documented that certain individuals are genetically predisposed to respond better to β-agonists, and in the next few years all of the remaining "asthma genes" should be discovered. Future treatments are likely to change the natural course of asthma.

At this time a number of new asthma medications are already in the "pipeline," moving toward regulatory approval. These medications will not eliminate the disease but should improve the quality of life of individuals with uncontrolled asthma.

New Medications

One entirely new family of asthma medication, phosphodiesterase4 inhibitors, should be available in the near future while further advances among existing medications are also forthcoming.

Phosphodiesterase4 Inhibitors

A new family of nonsteroidal anti-inflammatory medication known as phosphodiesterase4 (PDE4) inhibitors is under development for the treatment of asthma and chronic obstructive pulmonary disease (COPD). Roflumilast (Daxas) is a PDE4 inhibitor that has been shown to have broad anti-inflammatory effects. It is given orally and has been well tolerated. Clinical trials in people with asthma have shown benefits similar to those achieved with inhaled corticosteroids and anti-leukotrienes. Patients with asthma already receiving inhaled corticosteroids experienced further improvement when roflumilast was added to their regimen. This medication may be marketed first for the treatment of COPD.

Inhaled Corticosteroid: Ciclesonide

Ciclesonide (Alvesco) is a novel inhaled corticosteroid that is currently available for use in Europe, the United Kingdom, and South America. In clinical trials ciclesonide was shown to improve pulmonary function while reducing asthma symptoms and airway inflammation. This agent also appears to have no effect on adrenal function and may be administered once a day. When compared to other inhaled corticosteroids, ciclesonide may have fewer side effects.

Anti-Leukotrienes

Additional anti-leukotriene medications have yet to join montelukast, zafirlukast, and zileuton, which are currently in use in the United States. Pranukast (Onon) has been found to be as effective as montelukast but is not available in this country. An agent, MK-0591, which inhibits the action of an enzyme (5-lipoxygenase) involved in the formation of leukotrienes, has been found to be effective and appears promising. Verlukast, which blocks the action of leukotrienes after they are produced and may be given by inhalation, also appears to be effective but remains in development.

Mediator Antagonists

Asthma mediators are irritating chemicals that are either stored within allergy cells (mast cells, eosinophils) or produced when these cells are activated. These substances produce many changes that lead to inflammation of the bronchial tubes. Examples include histamine, leukotrienes, prostaglandins, cytokines (such as TNF-α), thromboxanes, and platelet-activating factor (PAF).

Thromboxane Antagonists. Seratrodast, a thromboxane antagonist, was the first drug of its kind approved for use (in Japan). The medication is given by mouth and has an excellent safety profile. Human studies to date, however, have shown a modest improvement in pulmonary function and asthma symptoms. At this time it is unclear as to whether this drug will be developed for the U.S. market. A second thromboxane antagonist, ramatroban, also has activity against prostaglandin D_2, which is a known bronchoconstrictor. This drug is also approved for use in Japan and has shown benefits in both allergic rhinitis and asthma. Clinical trials of ramatroban are under way in Europe.

Cytokines. Suplatast tosilate is a drug that inhibits several cytokines and is capable of reducing Immunoglobulin E (IgE) levels and numbers of eosinophils. One study in severe, steroid-dependent asthmatics found significant beneficial effects. Suplatast tosilate represents a novel and promising future treatment for asthma.

TNF-α Inhibitors. Inhibitors of TNF-α such as etanercept (Enbrel) were discussed in Chapter 4. Studies of these agents in patients with asthma are ongoing and are likely to produce results in the near future. TNF-α inhibitor therapy will likely be used in combination with standard stepwise therapy for selected patients with severe asthma.

Agent Combinations. Future development of mediator antagonists is also likely to produce combinations of more than one agent. One such medication under consideration is a combination of the anti-leukotriene, montelukast, and a prostaglandin D_2 inhibitor.

B_2-Agonists

Bambuterol (Bambec) is a drug that is converted by the body into another β_2-agonist, terbutaline. It is given by mouth and is effective for twenty-four hours. This once-a-day approach has proved helpful, especially for patients with nocturnal asthma. Bambuterol is available in Europe.

Xanthines

Xanthines belong to the medication group that contains theophylline. Two agents, doxofylline and enprofylline, have been studied and used in Europe. Doxofylline appears to have fewer side effects compared to theophylline and has been approved for use in Europe. The lower risk of adverse effects should reduce the need for blood level monitoring.

Future Uses of Omalizumab

In the next year omalizumab (Xolair) should be approved by the Food and Drug Administration for childhood asthma. In addition, it should become available in a pre-mixed, self-administered form. Approval may also be forthcoming for the use of omalizumab in allergic rhinitis, urticaria, eczema, and food allergies.

New Devices

Respimat Soft Mist Inhaler

A novel alternative to both metered-dose inhalers (MDIs) and dry powder inhalers (PDIs) is the Respimat device (Boehringer Ingelheim), which is currently available in Europe. This handheld, multidose device uses mechanical power from a spring rather than gas propellants to release doses of solutions for inhalation through a system of nozzles. Studies of this "soft mist" inhaler have revealed that it delivers greater lung deposition of medication compared to propellant MDIs and most DPIs. This device also does not require a forced inhalation and produces no irritation in the throat or mouth. The greater delivery of medication may also allow asthmatics to be treated with lower daily dosages of medication.

Combination Sprays

Symbicort. Symbicort, which combines the long-acting β_2-agonist formoterol with budesonide, an inhaled corticosteroid, should be released in the United States in 2007. This medication has been available in Europe in a multidose dry powder form but will be administered by an MDI in this country.

Berodual. Berodual combines a short-acting β_2-agonist, fenoterol, with ipratropium bromide, an anticholinergic bronchodilator. It is available in Europe and was the first aerosol made available with the Respimat Soft Mist Inhaler. At this time there are no plans to market this medication in the United States.

Advair HFA. Advair HFA combines the inhaled corticosteroid fluticasone with the long-acting β_2-agonist, salmeterol, in an MDI and should be available in this country in the near future. A multidose DPI, Advair Diskus, has been available for several years.

The Next Generation

Current asthma therapies have been shown to improve lung function, asthma symptoms, and quality of life, but none of these therapies prevents asthma or alters the long-term course of this disease. By targeting an individual's genetics, degree of airway irritability, and lung function, the next generation of asthma medications will most likely alter this course.

New medications will also provide more sustained relief of symptoms with fewer applications. Medications that are currently administered twice a day will likely be modified to once-a-day formulas. New combinations of medications are forthcoming and a three-drug medication (long-acting β_2-agonist, inhaled corticosteroid, and anticholinergic) for patients with mixed asthma and COPD is likely. New drugs such as the phosphodiesterase4 inhibitors will target inflammation and reduce airway narrowing. Additional antagonists of the chemical mediators of asthma such as suplatast will also be marketed and expanded use of TNF-α inhibitors in severe asthma is expected.

Over the next century, targeted asthma treatments will be developed that may possibly make asthma a disease of the past.

The Environment

Increased environmental controls over outdoor and indoor air pollution also will improve quality of life for the patient with bronchial asthma as well as the entire population. Federal guidelines for outdoor pollution have been established under the Clean Air Act amended in 1990. This act covers automobiles and industry and sets air quality standards that are regulated by the Environmental Protection Agency (EPA). Regional compliance with these standards has yet to be achieved, although progress has been made in some areas.

In many other areas, however, there is cause for concern. Modifications to the Clean Air Act in 2003 weakened regulation of dirty power plants, oil refineries, and other polluting facilities. These changes have been challenged in the courts but were recently partially upheld. In addition, despite a scientific consensus that air pollution standards need to be tightened to adequately protect the population, the EPA in December 2005 proposed new standards allowing higher pollution levels than the lowest levels recommended by their own scientists. Many individuals and groups, including the American Lung Association, have appealed this ruling.

Some states have passed laws with stricter standards that continue to tighten controls over automobile exhaust and the industrial combustion of fuels. Gasoline-engine manufacturers have reduced harmful emissions in their new vehicles by nearly 90 percent during the past thirty years, and makers of diesel engines have greatly reduced noxious exhaust fumes. Increased attention has also been directed at control of chlorofluorocarbon propellants that destroy the ozone layer. Although some progress has been made toward cleaner air, air pollution continues to be a major source of lung disease.

Greater attention must also be paid to "indoor pollution." This problem remains largely unregulated. Standards developed for outdoor pollution cannot be applied equally indoors. Fortunately, great strides have been made to restrict cigarette smoking. Further restrictions and ultimately a total ban on public smoking would be an important step toward reducing indoor and outdoor pollution as well as improving the general health of the entire population.

Every individual can be an active voice for improving the environment. Recent rulings relaxing or failing to tighten air pollution standards illustrate the need to press for true adherence to the Clean Air Act. Several organizations listed in the Appendix can provide further information on how to be heard at the local, state, and federal levels.

Forming a Partnership Against Asthma

Although medications are likely to be better in the future, patients must maintain an active role in preventing asthma attacks, particularly by avoiding and reducing irritants and allergens in their homes and work environments. If you have asthma, it is vital first to acknowledge that you have a problem and then to deal with it by working with your physician. Too often, denying the problem only leads to unnecessary illness. This first step may be the most important in a series of measures you can take to avoid asthma attacks.

Other measures include an "early warning system" that relies on home peak flow measurements and close communication between patients and their physicians to prevent serious and even potentially fatal attacks. Patient education should be given a high priority by physicians and their staffs. Self-education should always be encouraged. Through dialogue and education patients can recognize when they must call for assistance, thereby avoiding the life-threatening tendency to "push through" a serious asthma attack on their own.

This partnership between patients and physicians, both working toward reducing the frequency and severity of attacks, can succeed in improving the quality of life for those who have asthma. Cooperation can also reduce the number of fatal asthma attacks that often could have been prevented by earlier recognition and treatment of this largely reversible disease.

Appendix

How to Get More Help

By Phone

American Lung Association
800-LUNG USA (800-586-4872)

This toll-free number connects you to the local chapter of this national organization or to the national Lung HelpLine. Voice mail allows you to obtain information, order literature, and leave messages twenty-four hours a day. The Lung HelpLine provides the opportunity to speak to a lung health professional in English or Spanish who can help answer your lung health questions. It is available Monday through Friday, 7 a.m.–7 p.m. CST.

Asthma and Allergy Foundation of America (AAFA)
800-7-ASTHMA (800-727-8462)

The AAFA provides an information line to help consumers learn more about asthma and allergies, including referrals to physicians. The line is staffed Monday through Friday, 10 a.m.–3 p.m. EST.

National Jewish Medical and Research Center
800-222-LUNG (800-222-5864)

This information service is staffed by registered nurses who have been trained in respiratory, allergic, and immune diseases. They offer guidance by answering questions and providing educational materials, and if needed, referring callers to a National Jewish specialist. The service is available weekdays, 10 a.m.–6:30 p.m. EST.

Allergy and Asthma Supplies

Allergy Asthma Technology, Ltd.
8224 Lehigh Ave.
Morton Grove, IL 60053
800-621-5545; fax: 847-966-3068
allergyasthmatech.com

This is an informative company that provides a wide selection of allergy products. Their mail order catalog and Internet site include a selection of mattress and pillow covers, HEPA air filters, nebulizers, peak flow meters, and many other items as well as advice on allergy prevention. They have a pet section featuring Allerpet® Dander Solutions and other items including the Waterless Bath Pet Brush®. Their order form includes a "certificate of medical necessity" that may allow insurance reimbursement.

Allergy Control Products, Inc.
96 Danbury Rd.
Ridgefield, CT 06877
800-422-3878; fax: 203-431-8963
allergycontrol.com

This is a mail order company offering a comprehensive list of products incorporated into an educational brochure. Their products include pet allergy materials, several types of mattress and pillow covers, HEPA air filters, vacuum cleaners, and an allergy control video, available in English or in Spanish.

National Allergy Supply, Inc.
1600-D Satellite Blvd.
Duluth, GA 30097

800-522-1448; fax: 800-395-9303
natlallergy.com

This mail order company's allergy relief catalog offers many products for people with allergies, asthma, and sinus problems. Their catalog includes tips on controlling dust mites and comparison charts for HEPA vacuum cleaners and HEPA air cleaners. You may register for their monthly online newsletter.

American Lung Association Booklets and Fact Sheets

American Lung Association
61 Broadway, 6th Floor
New York, NY 10006
212-315-8700 (local) or 800-LUNG USA (800-586-4872);
    fax: 212-265-5642
lungusa.org

Booklets
Asthma Control Booklet—6 Steps (#2824)
Control Asthma—How to Recognize Asthma (#2827)
Teens and Asthma (#2832)

Fact Sheets
"Asthma" (#2834)
"Asthma at My Age" (#2829)
"Childhood Asthma" (#2825)
"Exercise and Lung Health" (#2844)
"Help Yourself to Better Breathing" (#2815)
"Home Control of Allergies and Asthma" (#2848)
"Indoor Air Pollution" (#2837)
"Outdoor Air Pollution" (#2835)
"Peak Flow Meters" (#2836)
"Radon" (#2841)
"Secondhand Smoke" (#2839)
"Tobacco Use" (#2840)

Many of the booklets and fact sheets are in Spanish as well as in English. The American Lung Association also has a Spanish section on its website.

Audiovisual Aids

Allergy Control Begins at Home
Publisher: Allergy Control Products, Inc.
96 Danbury Rd.
Ridgefield, CT 06877
800-422-3878; fax: 203-431-8963
allergycontrol.com

An informative video that describes the biology and living habits of dust mites and includes recommendations on how to decrease your level of exposure. It includes commentary by experts from the Asthma and Allergic Disease Center at the University of Virginia and is also available in Spanish.

Mastering Asthma
Publisher: Center for Children's Health Media
P.O. Box 269
Wilmington, DE 19899
888-440-2963
aquariusproductions.com

Produced by Nemours and the American Academy of Pediatrics, this video is designed to help families understand and live with childhood asthma.

Patient Education Videos and DVDs
Publisher: American Academy of Allergy, Asthma, and
    Immunology (AAAAI)
555 E. Wells St.
Milwaukee, WI 53202
414-272-6071; fax: 414-272-6070
aaaai.org

The videos available, including *Asthma and the Athlete*, provide an educational overview of asthma and allergies. Each video runs ten to thirteen minutes and may be purchased from the AAAAI.

Sit and Be Fit Videos
P.O. Box 8033
Spokane, WA 99203-0033
509-448-4938; fax: 509-448-5078
sitandbefit.com

Sit and Be Fit is a nonprofit organization committed to improving the quality of life of older adults, physically limited individuals, and those with chronic conditions through safe and effective exercises. Videos and DVDs may be purchased from their Internet site or by phone. Some cities have Sit and Be Fit exercise programs on television—check their Internet site for listings.

Books

Allergy Sourcebook, The. Maria Zellerbach. Chicago: McGraw-Hill, 2000 (304 pages). This book contains information on the types, triggers, and symptoms of allergy.

American Dietetic Association Complete Food and Nutrition Guide (2nd ed.). Roberta Larson Duyff. Hoboken, NJ: Wiley, 2002 (672 pages). A comprehensive guide to foods, nutrition, and diets, including the use and abuse of nutritional supplements.

American Lung Association Family Guide to Asthma and Allergies. Norman Edelman and the American Lung Association. Boston: Little, Brown, 1998 (256 pages). This book discusses the underlying causes of asthma and offers practical instructions on allergy proofing your home.

American Lung Association's 7 Steps to a Smoke-Free Life. Edwin B. Fisher. Hoboken, NJ: Wiley, 1998 (240 pages). This book presents information that will help you understand your smoking habit and offers a step-by-step approach to quitting.

Breathing Disorders Sourcebook, The. Francis V. Adams. Chicago: McGraw-Hill, 1998 (256 pages). How we breathe and what can go wrong are highlighted. This is an extensive guide to the causes, symptoms, and treatment of the most common types of breathing disorders.

Complete Food Allergy Cookbook. Marilyn Gioannini. Rocklin, CA: Prima Lifestyles, 1997 (336 pages). This cookbook has great recipes for special diets.

Coping with Prednisone. Eugenia Zukerman and Julie R. Ingelfinger. New York: St. Martin's Grifffin, 1998 (208 pages). This book discusses how to handle the side effects of oral corticosteroids, including recipes to avoid weight gain.

Exercises for Osteoporosis. Dianne Daniels. New York: Healthy Living Books, 2004 (160 pages). This book contains safe and effective exercises to build bone density and muscle strength in patients with this debilitating disease.

Harvard Medical School Guide to Healing Your Sinuses. Ralph Metson and Steven Mardon. Chicago: McGraw-Hill, 2005 (256 pages). This is a helpful guide to treating sinus disease.

How to Stop Heartburn: Simple Ways to Heal Heartburn and Acid Reflux. Anil Minocha and Christine Adamec. Hoboken, NJ: Wiley, 2001 (272 pages). This is a comprehensive book on treating heartburn and acid reflux.

Merck Manual of Health and Aging. Mark H. Beers (ed.). Whitehouse Station, NJ: Merck Laboratories, 2004 (961 pages). This helpful guide is about the changes and challenges of aging.

Merck Manual of Medical Information: Home Edition (2nd ed.). Mark H. Beers (ed.). Whitehouse Station, NJ: Merck Laboratories, 2004 (1,952 pages). This is the consumer-friendly version of the physician's *Merck Manual.*

My House Is Killing Me. Jeffrey C. May and Jonathan M. Samet. Baltimore: Johns Hopkins University Press, 2001 (400 pages). This is a useful guide for families with allergies and asthma.

PDR Pocket Guide to Prescription Drugs (7th ed.). P. D. R. Thompson. New York: Pocket, 2005 (1,760 pages). This guide contains brief and clearly written entries on major drugs and their side effects.

Positive Options for Children with Asthma. O. P. Jaggi. Alameda, CA: Hunter House, 2005 (164 pages). Information about childhood asthma is provided for parents.

Shortness of Breath: Guide to Better Living and Breathing (6th ed.). Andrew L. Ries, P. J. Bullock, W. D. Larsen, et al. St. Louis, MO: C.V. Mosby, 2000 (150 pages). This is a useful resource for patients with breathing disorders.

Sinus Sourcebook, The. Deborah Rosin. Chicago: McGraw-Hill, 1999 (208 pages). This book explains how the sinuses work and how to keep them healthy.

Strong Women, Strong Bones (rev. ed.). Miriam E. Nelson and Sarah Wernick. New York: Perigee Trade, 2001 (336 pages). This book offers suggestions on how to prevent and treat osteoporosis.

What Your Doctor May Not Tell You About Children's Allergies and Asthma. Paul Ehrlich and Larry Chiaramonte. Lebanon, IN: Warner Books, 2003 (336 pages). Simple steps are explained to help stop asthma attacks and improve your child's health.

Yoga Beats Asthma. Stella Weller. Toronto: HarperCollins Canada, 2003 (192 pages). Exercises and breathing techniques to help relieve asthma and respiratory disorders are included.

International Societies

Australian Lung Foundation (ALF)
Level 1,473 Lutwyche Rd.
P.O. Box 847
Lutwyche OLD 4030
800-654-301 (within Australia); fax: +61 (0)7 3357 6988
www.lungnet.org.au
e-mail: enquiries@lungnet.com.au

The Australian Lung Foundation is a not-for-profit public benevolent institution with medical and support group representation in every state and territory in Australia. It is the Australian counterpart to the American Lung Association.

Canadian Lung Association
3 Raymond St., Suite 300
Ottawa, ON KIR 1A3 Canada
613-569-6411; fax: 613-569-8860
lung.ca
e-mail: info@lung.ca

The Canadian Lung Association is the umbrella group for the ten provincial lung associations and is the Canadian counterpart to the American Lung Association. It provides information on asthma and other lung diseases in French as well as in English.

European Federation of Allergy and Airway Diseases (EFA)
Avenue Louise, 327
1050 Brussels
Belgium
+32 (0)2 646 9945; fax: +32 (0)2 646 4115
efanet.org
e-mail: info@efanet.org

The European Federation of Allergy and Airway Diseases supports the European network of professional national organizations. The central office of the EFA is located in Belgium.

National Societies

Allergy and Asthma Network/Mothers of Asthmatics, Inc.
  (AAN/MA)
2751 Prosperity Ave., Suite 150
Fairfax, VA 22031
800-878-4403; fax: 703-573-7794
aanma.org

Founded in 1985 by Nancy Sander, this health organization was originally Mothers of Asthmatics. The AAN/MA provides up-to-date information for patients and their families in English and in Spanish to promote a greater understanding of allergies and asthma. Membership includes subscriptions to *The MA Report* newsletter and *Allergy & Asthma Today* magazine as well as discounts on allergy and asthma products.

American Academy of Allergy, Asthma, and Immunology
  (AAAAI)
555 E. Wells St., Suite 1100
Milwaukee, WI 53202-3823
414-272-6071; fax: 414-272-6070
aaaai.org

This professional society of allergists and related specialists publishes the *Asthma and Allergy Advocate* for patients and the *Journal of Allergy and Clinical Immunology* for physicians. Patients may access the *Advocate*, pamphlets, and brochures from their website in English or in Spanish. For physician referrals, call 800-822-2762.

American Association for Respiratory Care (AARC)
9425 N. MacArthur Blvd., Suite 100
Irving, TX 75063-4706
972-243-2272; fax: 972-484-2720
aarc.org
e-mail: info@aarc.org

This professional society of respiratory therapists has a section dedicated to "Your Lung Health." Their Internet site includes an interactive movie about asthma in English and in Spanish.

American College of Allergy and Immunology (ACAAI)
85 W. Algonquin Rd., Suite 550
Arlington Heights, IL 60006
847-427-1200; fax: 847-427-1294
acaai.org
e-mail: Mail@acaai.org

This professional society of allergists and related specialists publishes the *Annals of Allergy and Immunology* for physicians and helps patients locate allergists. Allergy and asthma topics are in English and in Spanish.

American Dietetic Association (ADA)
120 S. Riverside Plaza, Suite 2000
Chicago, IL 60606-6995
800-877-1600; fax: 312-899-1979
eatright.org

The ADA and its National Center for Nutrition and Dietetics provide nutrition resources and the latest information on nutritional health. ADA's *Journal of the American Dietetic Association* (adajournal.org) is an important reference for the practice and science of nutrition.

American Lung Association
61 Broadway, 6th Floor
New York, NY 10006
212-315-8700; fax: 212-265-5642
lungusa.org

The American Lung Association is the leading organization working to prevent lung disease and promote lung health. This society publishes fact sheets and booklets in English and in Spanish. You may take the Asthma Control Test (asthmacontrol.com) in English or in Spanish, join an American Lung Association Freedom from Smoking® clinic, and subscribe to *Asthma Magazine* through their website.

American Thoracic Society (ATS)
61 Broadway
New York, NY 10006-2755
212-315-8700; fax: 212-315-6498
thoracic.org

The ATS is the medical branch of the American Lung Association (ALS). Besides many scientific activities, ATS/ALS has initiated the Asthma Research Campaign designed to promote multidisciplinary research aimed at producing a major advance in the prevention and treatment of asthma. The ATS also publishes the *American Journal of Respiratory and Critical Care Medicine*.

Asthma and Allergy Foundation of America (AAFA)
1233 20th St. NW, Suite 402
Washington, DC 20036
202-466-7643; fax: 202-466-8940
aafa.org
e-mail: info@aafa.org

The AAFA is a national organization sponsoring educational pro-grams for patients with asthma and allergies. The AAFA promotes research and asthma support groups. It also publishes the newslet-ter *Fresh Air* and the e-newsletter *Breathe* as well as educational material for children, teens, and schools in English and in Spanish. Each year the AAFA releases its "Asthma Capitals" list, a ranking of the 100 worst cities for asthma in the United States.

National Heart, Lung, and Blood Institute (NHLBI)
Information Center
P.O. Box 30105
Bethesda, MD 20824-0105
301-251-1222; fax: 240-629-3246
nhlbi.nih.gov
e-mail: nhlbiinfo@nhlbi.nih.gov

The NHLBI is the branch of the National Institutes of Health that sponsors cardiovascular and respiratory research and educational activities. Publications for the public include *Facts About Control-ling Your Asthma* in English and in Spanish.

National Institutes of Health (NIH)
9000 Rockville Pike
Bethesda, MD 20892
301-496-4000
nih.gov
e-mail: NIHinfo@od.nih.gov

The NIH is the U.S. government's major center for health research with links to its twenty-seven institutes and centers, including the National Institute of Allergy and Infectious Diseases and the National Library of Medicine.

U.S. Environmental Protection Agency (EPA)
Ariel Rios Building
1200 Pennsylvania Ave. NW
Washington, DC 20460
202-272-0167
epa.gov

The EPA was created in 1970 to promote a cleaner, healthier environment and is charged with carrying out the provisions of the Clean Air Act of 1990. You may contact the EPA for help with lead, radon, and other environmental hazards. Information is available in Spanish as well as in English.

U.S. Food and Drug Administration (FDA)
5600 Fishers Lane
Rockville, MD 20857
888-463-6332
www.fda.gov

The FDA regulates medicines, medical devices, foods, veterinary drugs, and many other products to ensure their safety and effectiveness. You may sign up for FDA's free e-mail newsletter and, if you wish, subscribe to the *FDA Consumer Magazine*, published bimonthly. The FDA's website has many fact sheets in Spanish as well as in English.

Newsletters and Magazines

Allergy & Asthma Today
Publisher: Allergy & Asthma Network Mothers of Asthmatics
2751 Prosperity Ave., Suite 150
Fairfax, VA 22031
800-878-4403; fax: 703-573-7794
breatherville.org

The official magazine of the Allergy & Asthma Network Mothers of Asthmatics published quarterly with the latest allergy and asthma news.

Consumer Reports on Health
Publisher: Consumer Union
101 Truman Ave.
Yonkers, NY 10703
consumerreports.org

Consumer Union publishes *Consumer Reports Magazine* as well as *Reports on Health* and *On Money*. If you have a subscription to a print newsletter, you have free access to their website.

Coping with Allergies and Asthma Magazine
Publisher: Media American Production, Inc.
P.O. Box 682268
Franklin, TN 37068-2268
615-791-3859; fax: 615-794-0179
copingmag.com

This consumer magazine is published five times a year with the latest asthma and allergy news.

Focus on Fitness Newsletter
Publisher: Sit and Be Fit
P.O. Box 8033
Spokane, WA 99203-0033
509-448-9438; fax: 509-448-5078
http://sitandbefit.com

Focus on Fitness is a twelve-page newsletter published in April and November containing educational articles covering fitness and healthy aging.

Harvard Health Publications
10 Shattuck St., Suite 612
Boston, MA 02115-6011
877-649-9457
health.harvard.edu

Harvard Health Publications, a division of Harvard Medical School, publishes five monthly newsletters: *Health, Heart, Mental Health, Women's Health Watch,* and *Men's Health Watch.* In addition to newsletters, Harvard Health Publications publishes Health Reports, including one on asthma and allergies.

Respiratory News & Views Newsletter
Publisher: Asthma/Emphysema Self-Help Group, Inc.
172 East 4th St., #11-F
New York, NY 10009
212-777-5581

This newsletter is published quarterly with the latest respiratory news and a listing of community support groups.

Second Wind Newsletter
Publisher: Pulmonary Education and Research Foundation
Pulmonary Education & Research Foundation
P.O. Box 1133
Lomita, CA 90717
310-539-8390
perf2ndwind.org

Second Wind is published nearly every month by the Pulmonary Education and Research Foundation (PERF). Most of the information in this newsletter can be viewed on the PERF website.

The Pulmonary Paper
Publisher: Self-published
Ormond Beach, FL 32175
386-673-5108
pulmonarypaper.org

This newsletter is published eight times a year and is dedicated to respiratory health care. Subscribers receive a 10 percent discount on items ordered from their respiratory recovery products.

UC Berkeley Wellness Letter
Publisher: University of California Berkeley
Subscription Dept.
P.O. Box 420148
Palm Coast, FL 32142
800-829-9170
wellnessletter.com

This is a monthly newsletter with information to promote and protect your health.

Referral Centers

The Nemours Institute–Alfred I. Dupont Hospital for Children
1600 Rockland Rd.
Wilmington, DE 19803
800-416-4441; fax: 302-651-6558
http://kidshealth.org

A comprehensive program for children with severe asthma that combines inpatient evaluation and outpatient therapy is offered.

National Jewish Medical and Research Center
1400 Jackson St.
Denver, CO 80206
800-222-5864
njc.org

This medical center is world renowned for its research, evaluation, and treatment of pulmonary diseases, including asthma. Patients of any age may be evaluated either as inpatients or as outpatients. Evaluations are thorough and combine several disciplines, including allergy, immunology, and pulmonology. Emphasis is placed on patient education and self-monitoring. Reports are sent promptly to referring physicians.

School Materials

Managing Asthma: A Guide for Schools
National Heart, Lung, and Blood Institute
Information Center
P.O. Box 30105
Bethesda, MD 20824-0105
301-592-8573; fax: 301-592-8563
nhlbi.nih.gov/health/public/lung/asthma/resolut.htm

The National Asthma Education and Prevention Program (NAEPP) for schools is coordinated by the National Heart, Lung, and Blood Institute.

Open Airways for Schools (OAS)
American Lung Association
61 Broadway, 6th Floor
New York, NY 10006
800-LUNG-USA
lungusa.org

Open Airways for Schools consists of six 40-minute group lessons for children with asthma held during the school day. *OAS* uses group discussion, stories, games, and role play to help students take part in the program. Instructors are trained in the program by a certified trainer. Instructors can be school personnel, parents, community volunteers, or anyone with an interest in working with children. *OAS* is provided to the school or school district by local lung associations or partner organizations.

Support Groups

American Lung Association
61 Broadway, 6th Floor
New York, NY 10006
212-315-8700; fax: 212-265-5642
lungusa.org

For information on the American Lung Association's Better Breathers Clubs in your area, log on to the American Lung Association's website or call 800-LUNG-USA (800-586-4872).

Asthma and Allergy Foundation of America (AAFA)
1233 20th St. NW, Suite 402
Washington, D.C. 20036
202-466-8940; fax: 202-466-8940
aafa.org

The AAFA offers a free subscription to *Leaders Link*, a group leader/advisor newsletter. The educational support group section of AAFA's website helps you find a group in your area and also tells you how to start a group that would be affiliated with AAFA.

Asthma/Emphysema Self-Help Groups
172 East 4th St., Apt. 11F
New York, NY 10009
212-330-7894

This organization consists of Manhattan-based self-help groups. Call for locations and for information about self-help groups in other areas.

On the Internet

Allergy and Asthma Supplies

Allergy Asthma Technology, Ltd.
allergyasthmatech.com

Allergy Control Products, Inc.
allergycontrol.com

National Allergy Supply, Inc.
natlallergy.com

Audiovisual Aids

Allergy Control Begins at Home
allergycontrol.com

Mastering Asthma
aquariusproductions.com

Asthma Triggers
Asthma Management
Asthma and the Athlete
aaaai.org

Sit and Be Fit
sitandbefit.com

International Societies

Australian Lung Foundation (ALF)
lungnet.org.au

Canadian Lung Association
lung.ca

European Federation of Allergy and Airway Diseases (EFA)
efanet.org

National Societies

Allergy and Asthma Network/Mothers of Asthmatics, Inc. (AANMA)
aanma.org

American Academy of Allergy, Asthma, and Immunology (AAAAI)
aaaai.org

American Association for Respiratory Care (AARC)
aarc.org

American College of Allergy, Asthma, and Immunology (ACAAI)
acaai.org

American Dietetic Association (ADA)
eatright.org

American Lung Association
lungusa.org

American Thoracic Society (ATS)
thoracic.org

Asthma and Allergy Foundation of America (AAFA)
aafa.org

National Heart, Lung, and Blood Institute (NHLBI)
nhlbi.nih.gov

National Institutes of Health (NIH)
nih.gov

U.S. Environmental Protection Agency (EPA)
epa.gov

U.S. Food and Drug Administration (FDA)
fda.gov

Newsletters/Magazines

Allergy & Asthma Today
breatherville.org

Asthma Magazine
elsevierhealth.com

Consumer Reports on Health
consumerreports.org

Coping with Allergies and Asthma
copingmag.com

Focus on Fitness Newsletter
http://sitandbefit.com

Harvard Health Publications
health.harvard.edu

The Pulmonary Paper
pulmonarypaper.org

Second Wind Newsletter
perf2ndwind.org

UC Berkeley Wellness Letter
wellnessletter.com

Referral Centers

The Nemours Institute—Alfred I. Dupont Hospital for Children
http://kidshealth.org

National Jewish Medical and Research Center
njc.org

School Materials

Managing Asthma: A Guide for Schools
nhlbi.nih.gov/health/public/lung/asthma/resolut.htm

Open Airways for Schools
alany.org/oas.html

Support Groups

American Lung Association
lungusa.org

Asthma and Allergy Foundation of America (AAFA)
aafa.org

General Health Information

American Kennel Club (AKC)
akc.org

The AKC provides detailed descriptions of 150 breeds and lists those that are less likely to produce an allergic reaction. The website also includes referrals to breeders.

Ask Noah
noah-health.org

This site provides New York online access to health information in either English or in Spanish.

The Breathing Source
adamsmd.com

This news page provides current information on asthma with links to informative health sites.

Aetna InteliHealth, Inc.
http://intelihealth.com

Features Harvard Medical School's Consumer Health Information, a vast resource of medical information.

Clarinex
allergy-relief.com

This website provides allergy news and allows you to register for an electronic newsletter with local pollen counts.

Just Move
justmove.org

The American Heart Association's Fitness Center provides fitness resources and recommendations for achieving the greatest benefit from physical activity.

Mayo Clinic
mayoclinic.com

Access health information from the Mayo Clinic. This website offers free subscription to *Housecall*, a weekly e-newsletter.

Medline Plus
http://medlineplus.gov

This website contains information from the National Library of Medicine, including clinical trials, a medical encyclopedia, and links to other sites including NIH SeniorHealth.

Merck Source
mercksource.com

Learn about your condition and find help and support from this site. Register to receive a monthly *Source Report* newsletter on a number of topics including allergy and asthma.

MyAsthma
myasthma.com

This site is designed to assist you in managing your asthma and allergies through online forums. You can track your peak flow and review your progress with graphs and reports that may be shared with your health-care provider.

NYU Medical Center
med.nyu.edu

This award-winning website includes links to NYU's world-renowned Rusk Institute of Rehabilitation Medicine.

No Air to Go
http://noairtogo.tripod.com

This website contains a glossary of pulmonary definitions with a quick reference to pulmonary function testing.

Weather Channel
weather.com/health

Information on asthma and allergies with countrywide allergy maps based on weather and pollen counts can be found on this website.

WebMD
http://webmd.com

A to Z Health Guides, latest news, and weekly and biweekly newsletters on topics of interest are available.

Your Lung Health
yourlunghealth.org

Sponsored by the American Association for Respiratory Care, this website offers information about diseases of the lungs.

Prescription Medications

U.S. Food and Drug Administration (FDA)
fda.gov

The FDA regulates medicine, medical devices, foods, veterinary drugs, and many other products to ensure their safety and effectiveness. This website can also be used to research the products the FDA regulates.

RX List-Internet Drug Index
rxlist.com

This easy-to-use website can be used to research medications. It also provides links to numerous health-related sites.

Search Engines

Google
google.com

This is a general search engine.

Healthfinder
healthfinder.gov

This is a service of the National Health Information Center with consumer health information from federal organizations and a health library from A to Z. This website is in English and in Spanish.

Yahoo! Health
http://dir.yahoo.com/health

This popular search engine offers the latest health information on a full range of topics.

Glossary

Acaracide—agent that can be used in the home to eradicate dust mites

Acetylcholine—chemical substance, stored in nerve endings of the parasympathetic nervous system, released when nerves are stimulated, producing a response

Adrenergic—refers to sympathetic nervous system and its nerve fibers and receptors. Stimulating these receptors in the bronchial tubes produces bronchial muscle relaxation, resulting in opening of the bronchial tubes.

Aerosol—fine mist that can be inhaled; may be produced by metered-dose inhaler or nebulizer

Agonist—drug or agent with an affinity for corresponding nerve receptor that may stimulate the receptor to produce its effect. For example, a beta-agonist attaches to a beta-receptor, producing relaxation of bronchial lining muscle.

Airway hyperreactivity—asthma characteristic in which bronchial tubes react to substances or stimuli by closing or constricting, a reaction that does not occur in nonasthmatics

Allergen—substance producing allergic reaction, for example, airborne pollen

Allergy—hypersensitivity to a specific substance. When an allergic person is exposed to an offending substance, a "reaction" occurs that may take several forms (tearing of eyes, sneezing, wheezing) varying from person to person.

Alveoli—tiny air sacs that make up lung tissue where the exchange of oxygen and carbon dioxide occurs

Anaphylaxis—extremely severe allergic reaction involving the total body, often characterized by "closing" of the throat and constriction of bronchial tubes. May result in collapse of body's circulation (shock) and death.

Atelectasis—lung condition in which tiny air sacs or alveoli are collapsed

Atopy—condition of being allergic; often used interchangeably with *allergy*

Autonomic nervous system—the body's involuntary control system that maintains many functions; divided into parasympathetic and sympathetic branches

Beta-agonist—medication-stimulating nerve receptors that produce bronchial tube dilatation

Beta-receptor—nerve-ending site responsible for bronchial tube condition

Bronchial tubes—air passages of the lung through which air exchange takes place. The asthmatic reaction takes place in these tubes.

Bronchiectasis—condition in which infection has damaged the bronchial tube wall, producing chronic cough and production of infected sputum. Wheezing may also occur during this condition, which may be confused with asthma.

Bronchoconstriction—narrowing or closing of bronchial tubes; one characteristic of an asthmatic reaction

Bronchodilatation—opening or widening of bronchial tubes; reverse of *bronchoconstriction*

Bronchodilator—agent or medication producing bronchodilatation

Bronchoscopy—procedure in which a lighted scope called a bronchoscope is introduced into lungs through bronchial tubes. It is usually done to investigate certain lung diseases.

Bronchospasm—the narrowing of bronchial airways; same as *bronchoconstriction*

Candidiasis—fungal infection caused by the common yeast *Candida*. It may occur in the mouth in patients with poor oral hygiene who use corticosteroid sprays and may be prevented with simple precautions and treated with anti-fungal medication.

Capillaries—tiny blood vessels found in walls of alveoli in lung and other parts of the body. In the lung, these vessels pick up oxygen and release carbon dioxide.

Carbon dioxide (CO_2)—waste product of body metabolism; gas excreted by lung in exhalation

CFCs—abbreviation for *chlorofluorocarbons*; chemical aerosols currently powering metered-dose inhalers. Known to be harmful to the ozone layer.

Cholinergic—related to stimulation of the parasympathetic nervous system. In the lung this causes contraction of bronchial muscle, producing bronchoconstriction.

Chromosome—structure within body cells that contains genes

Corticosteroid—group of medications derived from adrenal gland

Cystic fibrosis—hereditary childhood lung disease characterized by cough, thick mucus, and recurrent lung infections. Wheezing may also occur and cause confusion with asthma diagnosis.

DPI—abbreviation for *dry powder inhaler*

Emphysema—lung disease in which walls of air sacs are destroyed and supporting structure of bronchial tubes is weakened. Emphysema may be confused with asthma due to presence of wheezing.

Endoscope—flexible, lighted instrument for examining internal organs. See also *bronchoscopy.*

Eosinophil—a white blood cell associated with allergic reactions; often involved in asthma.

Ergometer—instrument for measuring amount of work or energy the body uses.

Expiratory—relating to breathing out, or exhaling

Fiberoptic—fine glass fibers that transmit images in instruments for examining internal organs (endoscopes)

Freon—see *CFCs*

Gastroesophageal—relating to the upper digestive system, including feeding passage (esophagus) and stomach

HFA—abbreviation for *hydrofluoroalkane*, a non-CFC chemical propellant for metered-dose inhalers

High-efficiency particulate air purifier (HEPA)—filters that can be used in room air purifiers, central ventilation systems, and vacuum cleaners

Histamine—chemical substance contained in MAST cells and other white blood cells. When histamine is released from these cells, it may cause many features of allergic reaction.

Humidification—addition of moisture to air. May be used to loosen dried secretions in sinuses or bronchial tubes.

Humoral—relating to the substance produced in the body that acts at a specific site, for example, production of antibodies by the immune system

Hyperinflated—lung condition in which lungs are overexpanded; may occur in asthma when inhaled air is "trapped" by narrowed bronchial tubes

Hyperreactivity—condition of increased sensitivity or irritability, a feature of bronchial tubes in asthma

Hyperresponsiveness—see *hyperreactivity*

Immunoglobulin—protein substance produced by immune system in response to body being invaded by foreign substance (allergen or bacteria). Several types are produced depending on the invader.

Immunoglobulin E (IgE)—a type of immunoglobulin produced when sensitive individual is exposed to allergens. Blood levels of IgE may identify presence of allergy in some individuals. Immunoglobulin E is involved in allergic reaction that allows allergy chemicals to be released from storage cells.

Immunotherapy—allergy treatment also known as "desensitization" or "allergy shots." Injections of extracts of allergy substances are given in increasing strengths over time.

Intranasal—refers to application of medication into nasal passages

Intravenous—injecting medication directly into a vein

Intubation—placing breathing tube into the windpipe, performed when artificial or mechanical respiration is needed

Lymphocyte—white blood cell commonly involved in immune reactions. T lymphocytes are involved in cellular reactions; B lymphocytes are responsible for production of antibodies.

Mast cells—body cells that contain chemicals that are mediators of asthma and allergy reactions. These cells are distributed throughout the body and are commonly found on the surfaces of the nose, throat, and bronchial tubes. When these cells are destroyed, their chemical contents are released and allergy and asthma reactions occur.

Mediator—chemical substance that produces a body reaction when released

Metered-dose inhaler (MDI)—handheld applicator that dispenses liquid asthma medication in an aerosol medium for inhalation

Methacholine—cholinergic drug that may produce broncho-constriction when administered to asthmatics. Often used in bronchial challenge testing to demonstrate presence or absence of reactive airways.

Mucosa—mucous membrane covering inner surface of many structures in the body, including the nose and bronchial tubes. This delicate bronchial lining swells and becomes inflamed in an asthmatic attack.

Myopathy—muscle abnormality possibly characterized by weakness and atrophy. Potential adverse effect of systemic corticosteroids

Nebulizer—device that dispenses liquid medication as a fine mist that is inhaled. Devices vary in the size of particles they dispense.

Neurotransmitter—chemical substance that facilitates conduction of nerve impulses

Neutrophil—type of white blood cell often involved in immune reactions

NSAID—abbreviation for *nonsteroidal anti-inflammatory drug*

Ostia—openings in various canals or tubes throughout body; for example, nasal and sinus passages

Over-the-counter (OTC) medications—medications that do not need a physician's prescription to be sold

Oximeter—device measuring saturation or enrichment of blood with oxygen

Oxygen—gas needed for life-sustaining activities of body; taken up by red blood cells within walls of alveoli

Particulates—fine airborne particles (soot) produced by fuel combustion; a component of air pollution

Polypectomy—surgical procedure to remove polyps from various body locations including nose and sinuses. Recent advances in technology may allow polyp removal by endoscopic surgery.

Prokinetic—characteristic of certain medications that increase forward motility of digestive tract. May be used to treat gastroesophageal reflux.

Pulmonologist—internist with specialized training in lung diseases. After completing required training, physician may take certifying examination in pulmonary disease given by American Board of Internal Medicine.

Racemic—man-made, as opposed to a chemical naturally produced in the body

Radioallergosorbent test (RAST)—a blood test that can identify allergy to specific substances; an alternative to allergy scratch tests; measures amount of IgE manufactured by body against specific allergens

Reflux—backward flow; a term commonly describing regurgitation of stomach contents into feeding passage (esophagus)

Rhinitis—inflammation of nasal membranes or lining; may be allergic or nonallergic

Scratch test—allergy test in which the skin is scratched and a drop of allergen is placed on scratched area. An alternative is the prick test, in which an allergen is placed on the skin, which is pricked with a needle.

Spirometer—instrument used to measure air capacity of lungs; may also be equipped to measure speed of air movement

Spirometry—testing with spirometer; may be called "pulmonary function test"

Sputum—material coughed up from lungs; also *phlegm*; consists of mucus, cells, and debris resulting from bacteria

Symptomatology—aggregate of symptoms from disease

Systemic—term referring to the entire body. Often describes how a medication is given; in contrast to "local" medication given at specific site, systemic drugs are taken by mouth or intravenously and pass through entire body.

Tomography—x-ray technique allowing sections of a structure to be visualized in detail

Trachea—main air passage or windpipe beginning below voice box (larynx) and ending when it divides into the right and left main bronchial tubes. Trachea is considered one of the "large airways."

Urticaria—skin eruption of hives; usually represents a systemic allergic reaction

Vagus—major nerve with parasympathetic (cholinergic) fibers distributed to bronchial tubes. Stimulating these nerves may cause constriction of bronchial tubes. Anticholinergic medications that block vagal impulses may be bronchodilatators.

Bibliography

Adams, F.V. *The Breathing Disorders Sourcebook*. Chicago: McGraw-Hill, 1998.

———. *Healing Through Empathy*. New York: iUniverse, 2004.

Agata, H., A. Yomo, Y. Hanashiro, et al. 1993. "Comparison of the MAST Chemiluminescent Assay System with RAST and Skin Tests in Allergic Children." *Annals of Allergy*, 70:153–157.

Anderson, S.D., L.T. Rodwell, J. Du Toit, and I.H. Young. 1991. "Duration of Protection by Inhaled Salmeterol in Exercise-Induced Asthma." *Chest*, 100:1254–1260.

Ballard, R.D. 1994. "Nocturnal Asthma: Potential Mechanisms and Current Therapy." *Clinical Pulmonary Medicine*, 1(5):271–278.

Barnes, P.J. 1989. "A New Approach to the Treatment of Asthma." *The New England Journal of Medicine*, 321:517–527.

———. 1994. "Blunted Perception and Death from Asthma." *The New England Journal of Medicine*, 330:1383–1384.

Barnes, P.J., K.F. Chung, T.W. Evans, and S.G. Spiro. *Therapeutics in Respiratory Disease*. Edinburgh: Churchill Livingstone, 1994.

Barnes, P.J., S. Pedersen, and W.W. Busse. 1998. "Efficacy and Safety of Inhaled Corticosteroids. New Developments."

Respiratory and Critical Care Medicine, 157 (Supplement): S1–S53.

Becket, W.S. 2000. "Occupational Respiratory Diseases." *The New England Journal of Medicine*, 342(6):406–413.

Bernstein, I.L. 1981. "Occupational Asthma." *Clinics in Chest Medicine*, 2(2):255–272.

Bevelaqua, F.A., and F.V. Adams. 2005. "Pulmonary Disorders." In Eisenberg, M.G., E.F. Richter, and H.H. Zaretsky (eds): *Medical Aspects of Disability*, 3rd ed. (543–563). New York: Springer.

Blanc, P.D. 1993. "Work Disability Among Adults with Asthma." *Chest*, 104:1371–1377.

Britton, J., I. Pavord, K. Richards, et al. 1994. "Dietary Magnesium, Lung Function, Wheezing, and Airway Hyperreactivity in a Random Adult Population Sample." *Lancet*, 344:357–362.

Burrows, B., and M.D. Lebowitz. 1992. "The B-Agonist Dilemma." *The New England Journal of Medicine*, 326:560–561.

Check, W.A., and M. Kaliner. 1990. "Pharmacology and Pharmokinetics of Topical Corticosteroid Derivatives Used for Asthma Therapy." *American Review of Respiratory Disease*, 141:S44–S51.

Considerations for Diagnosing and Managing Asthma in the Elderly. 1996. Washington, D.C.: U.S. Dept. of Health and Human Services (NAEPP Working Group Report). NIH Pub. No. 96-3662.

Cooke, J.R. 2005. "Emerging Concepts for Understanding Asthma." *The Respiratory Report*, 1(1):18–25.

Corren, J., R. Berkowitz, J.J. Murray, et al. 2003. "Comparison of Once-Daily Mometasone Furoate Versus Once-Daily Budesonide in Patients with Moderate Persistent Asthma." *International Journal of Clinical Practice*, 57(7):567–572.

D'Alonzo, G.E., S.I. Rennard, P.R. Ratner, and S.R. Findlay. 1992. "Twice-Daily Inhaled Salmeterol as Maintenance Therapy for Asthma." *American Review of Respiratory Disease*, 145(4, pt. 2): Abstract 65.

Dolovich, M., R. Ruffin, D. Corr, and M.T. Newhouse. 1983. "Clinical Evaluation of a Simple Demand Inhalation MDI Aerosol Delivery Device." *Chest*, 84:36–41.

Engleberg, A. *The Respiratory System: Guides to the Evaluation of Permanent Impairment.* Chicago: American Medical Association, 1988.

Erzurum, S.C. 2006. "Inhibition of Tumor Necrosis Factor α for Refractory Asthma." *The New England Journal of Medicine*, 354(7):754–758.

Fiore, M.C., L.J. Baker, and S.M. Deeren. 1993. "Cigarette Smoking: The Leading Preventable Cause of Pulmonary Diseases." In Bone, R.C. (ed): *Pulmonary and Critical Care Medicine.* St. Louis: Mosby.

Glassberg, A. 2005. "Emerging Concepts in Asthma: Inflammation, Disease Modification, and the Role of IgE." *The Respiratory Report*, 1(2):5–13.

Grossman, J. 1994. "The Evolution of Inhaler Technology." *Journal of Asthma*, 31(1):55–64.

Guidelines for the Diagnosis and Management of Asthma. 1991. Washington, D.C.: U.S. Dept. of Health and Human Services (National Asthma Education Program). NIH Pub. No. 91-3042.

Guidelines for the Diagnosis and Management of Asthma—Update on Selected Topics 2002. 2003. Washington, D.C.: U.S. Dept. of Health and Human Services (NAEPP Expert Panel Report). NIH Pub. No. 02-5075.

Haahtela, T., M. Jarvinen, T. Kava, et al. 1994. "Effects of Reducing or Discontinuing Inhaled Budesonide in Patients with Mild Asthma." *The New England Journal of Medicine*, 331:700–705.

Haas, F., S. Pasierski, N. Levine, et al. 1987. "Effect of Aerobic Training on Forced Expiratory Airflow in Exercising Asthmatic Humans." *Journal of Applied Physiology*, 63:1230–1235.

Hampson, N.B., and M.P. Mueller. 1994. "Reduction in Patient Timing Errors Using a Breath-Activated Metered-Dose Inhaler." *Chest*, 106(2):462–465.

Horwitz, R.J., K.A. McGill, and W.W. Busse. 1998. "The Role of Leukotriene Modifiers in the Treatment of Asthma." *Respiratory and Critical Care Medicine*, 157:1363–1371.

International Consensus Report on Diagnosis and Treatment of Asthma. 1992. Washington, D.C.: U.S. Dept. of Health and Human Services (International Asthma Management Project). NIH Pub. No. 92-3091.

Janson, C., E. Bjornsson, J. Hetta, et al. 1994. "Anxiety and Depression in Relation to Respiratory Symptoms and Asthma." *American Journal of Respiratory and Critical Care Medicine*, 149:930–934.

Johansson, S.A., K.E. Andersson, R. Brattsand, et al. 1982. "Topical and Systemic Glucocorticoid Potencies of Budesonide and Beclomethasone Dipropionate in Man." *European Journal of Clinical Pharmacology*, 22:523–529.

Kikuchi, Y., S. Okabe, G. Tamura, et al. 1994. "Chemosensitivity and Perception of Dyspnea in Patients with a History of Near-Fatal Asthma." *The New England Journal of Medicine*, 330:1329–1334.

Konig, P. 1988. "Inhaled Corticosteroids—Their Present and Future Role in the Management of Asthma." *The Journal of Allergy and Clinical Immunology*, 82(2):297–306.

Leath, T.M., M. Singla, and S.P. Peters. 2005. "Novel and Emerging Therapies for Asthma." *Drug Discovery Today*, 10(23/24):1647–1655.

Lee, D., T. Fardon, C. Bates, et al. 2005. "Airway and Systemic Effects of Hydrofluoroalkane Formulations of High-Dose Ciclesonide and Fluticasone in Moderate Persistent Asthma." *Chest*, 127:851–860.

Lee, N., G. Rachelefsky, R.H. Kobayashi, et al. 1991. "Efficacy and Safety of Albuterol Administered by Power-Driven Nebulizer (PDN) Versus Metered-Dose Inhaler (MDI) with Aerochamber and Mask in Infants and Young Children with Acute Asthma." *Journal of Allergy and Clinical Immunology*, 87(Suppl.)(1, pt. 2):307.

Lung Disease Data 1997. 1997. New York: American Lung Association.

Management of Asthma During Pregnancy. 1993. Washington, D.C.: U.S. Dept. of Health and Human Services (Report of the Working Group on Asthma and Pregnancy). NIH Pub. No. 93-3279A.

Managing Asthma During Pregnancy: Recommendations for Pharmacologic Treatment. 2004. Washington, D.C.: U.S. Dept. of Health and Human Services. NIH Pub. No. 05-3279.

Martinez, F.D. 2005. "Safety of Long-Acting Beta-Agonists—An Urgent Need to Clear the Air." *The New England Journal of Medicine*, 353(25):2637–2639.

McKeever, T.M., and J. Britton. 2004. "Diet and Asthma." *American Journal of Respiratory and Critical Care Medicine*, 170:725–729.

Nelson, H.S. 2006. "Is There a Problem with Inhaled Long-Acting Beta-Adrenergic Agonists?" *Journal of Allergy and Clinical Immunology*, 117(1):3–16.

Newhouse, M.T. 1993. "Pulmonary Drug Targeting with Aerosols. Principles and Clinical Applications in Adults and Children." *The American Journal of Asthma & Allergy for Pediatricians*, 7(1):23–35.

Newman, S.P., J. Brown, K.P. Steed, et al. 1998. "Lung Deposition of Fenoterol and Flunisolide Delivered Using a Novel Device for Inhaled Medicines." *Chest*, 113:957–963.

Newman, S.P., G. Woodman, S.W. Clarke, and M.A. Sackner. 1986. "Effect of InspirEase on the Deposition of Metered-Dose Aerosols in the Human Respiratory Tract." *Chest*, 89:551–556.

O'Byrne, P.M., I. Israel, and J.M. Drazen. 1997. "Anti-Leukotrienes in the Treatment of Asthma." *Annals of Internal Medicine*, 127:472–480.

O'Riordan, T.G., W. Mao, L.B. Palmer, et al. 2006. "Assessing the Effects of Racemic and Single-Enantiomer Albuterol on Airway Secretions in Long-Term Intubated Patients." *Chest*, 129(1):124–132.

Otsuka, K.N. 2005. "Advances in Asthma Pharmacotherapy over the Past 100 Years." *The Respiratory Report*, 1(2):14–21.

Pearlman, D.S., P. Chervinsky, C. Laforce, et al. 1992. "A Comparison of Salmeterol with Albuterol in the Treatment of Mild-to-Moderate Asthma." *The New England Journal of Medicine*, 327:1420–1425.

Penvenne, L.J. 1997. "High-Tech Help for Dirty Diesels." *Technology Review*, 1:2.

Petrie, G.R. 1993. "Bambuterol: Effective in Nocturnal Asthma." *Respiratory Medicine*, 87:581–585.

Rau, Jr., J.L. *Respiratory Care Pharmacology*. St. Louis: Mosby, 1994.

Samet, J.M., and M.J. Utell. 1993. "Air Pollution." In Bone, R.C. (ed): *Pulmonary and Critical Care Medicine*. St. Louis: Mosby.

Shirakawa, T., L. Airong, M. Dubowitz, et al. 1994. "Association Between Atopy and Variants of the B Subunit of the High-Affinity Immunoglobulin E Receptor." *Nature Genetics*, 7(2):125–129.

Sorkness, R., J.J. Clough, W.L. Castleman, and R.F Lemanske, Jr. 1994. "Virus-Induced Airway Obstruction and Parasympathetic Hyperresponsiveness in Adult Rats." *American Journal of Respiratory and Critical Care Medicine*, 150:28–34.

Spector, S.L., L.J. Smith, M. Glass, et al. 1994. "Effect of Six Weeks of Therapy with Oral Doses of ICI 204,219, a Leukotriene D_4 Receptor Antagonist in Subjects with Bronchial Asthma." *American Journal of Respiratory and Critical Care Medicine*, 150:618–623.

Spitzer, W.O., S. Suissa, P. Ernst, et al. 1992. "The Use of B-Agonists and the Risk of Death and Near Death from Asthma." *The New England Journal of Medicine*, 326:502–506.

Thompson, J., T. Irvine, K. Grathwohl, and B. Roth. 1994. "Misuse of Metered-Dose Inhalers in Hospitalized Patients." *Chest*, 105(3):715–717.

Turkeltaub, P.C. 1994. "Deaths Associated with Allergenic Extracts." *FDA Medical Bulletin*, 24(1):7.

Vanzieleghem, M.A., and E.F. Juniper. 1987. "A Comparison of Budesonide and Beclomethasone Dipropionate Nasal Aerosols in Ragweed-Induced Rhinitis." *Journal of Allergy and Clinical Immunology*, 79:887–892.

Weiss, K.B., P.J. Gergen, and T.A. Hodgson. 1992. "An Economic Evaluation of Asthma in the United States." *The New England Journal of Medicine*, 326:862–866.

Ziment, I. 1995. "Alternative Medicine and Asthma." *Pulmonary Perspectives*, 12:1–3.

Index

Page numbers followed by *f* or *t* refer to figures or tables respectively.